COACHING CHILDREN

SPORTS SCIENCE ESSENTIALS

—— Kelly Sumich ——

ACER Press

RICH AU

First published 2013
by ACER Press, an imprint of
Australian Council *for* Educational Research Ltd
19 Prospect Hill Road, Camberwell
Victoria, 3124, Australia

www.acerpress.com.au
sales@acer.edu.au

Edited by Elisa Webb
Cover design, text design and typesetting by ACER Project Publishing

Printed in Australia by McPherson's Printing Group

National Library of Australia Cataloguing-in-Publication data:

Author: Sumich, Kelly, author.

Title: Coaching children : sports science essentials / Kelly Sumich.

ISBN: 9781742860626 (paperback)

Notes: Includes bibliographical references.

Subjects: Sports for children--Coaching.
                 Coaching (Athletics)
                 Physical education and training.
                 Sports sciences.

Dewey Number: 613.7042

DISCLAIMER

The information in this book is proffered as helpful and informative material on the
subject of coaching children in sport. It is not in any way intended to supplement or replace
professional medical or sports science advice. The author, editor and publisher make no
warranties whatsoever, express or implied, with respect to any material contained in the
book and specifically disclaim any liability arising directly or indirectly from use of the book.

PEFC is committed to sustainable forest management
through third party forest certification.
For more information go to www.pefc.org

FOREWORD

Sport has long been described as an essential part of Australian culture and approximately seven in ten children participate in sporting activities outside of school hours. Young people like to play sport as it gives them an opportunity to have fun with their friends and experience enjoyment, achieve goals and develop game skills. However, many factors conspire against healthy sports participation rates over the longer term. The cost of uniforms, registration fees and treating sports injuries, or other pressures such as competing obligations, transport issues and busy family life can all affect adherence rates.

Many of these factors are outside of the coach's influence, but there some reasons that children drop out which you can help to remedy, such as children becoming bored with a sport, children not getting enough playing time on the field or too much emphasis being placed on winning. You have a most important role in children's sport; as a coach, you are responsible for dealing with athletes who are rapidly growing and developing. It is of upmost importance that you ensure all athletes in your care gain optimum benefit and enjoyment from sports participation and that children's physical, social and mental needs are catered for in a professional manner. A coach must treat all players equally, yet treat each athlete as an individual; they need to acknowledge the contribution of all team members and design safe, fun and friendly training programs.

Coaching children: sports science essentials has been written to provide essential information about coaching children in sport. It has been specifically targeted to help the parents and coaches throughout Australia who wish to build their knowledge and awareness of sports science and improve their coaching. Kelly Sumich's book is organised into seven key chapters. Chapter 1 discusses the development of children's sports skills. Kelly notes in this chapter how motor skill development is essential in providing the basic foundations for a child to perform in sport. Recent research shows that standards are slipping and children need to be taught the correct way to perform these skills. This chapter also demonstrates for the reader how to structure sports training to suit children's individual skill levels.

In Chapter 2, you can learn about designing safe programs to cater for children's physical and social development. This chapter addresses how you can set your expectations and training goals to suit children's performance capabilities, in contrast to those designed for adults. Chapter 3 hones in on important fitness principles and those elements to consider when designing an effective training program to prepare children for competition. Chapter 4 focuses on the communication skills such as feedback and active listening. It also provides an outline for achieving longevity in sport, of the importance of children's 'developmental age' and related influences on participation and specialisation in a sport.

Chapter 5 explains how you can motivate children and assist them to develop a positive attitude towards sports and exercise. Most appropriately, it also covers techniques to manage anxiety, set goals, keep winning in perspective and help children cope with competition. Chapter 6 explains food nutrients and fluid intakes so that you understand how these can be used to help promote sports performance. The final chapter of the book provides information on how you can create safe training programs and environments to avoid athletic injury. A background to common sporting injuries and their treatment follows, to aid injured children's safe return to sport.

'Reflective questions for the coach' contained at the end of every chapter will help to make sure that you gain the most from the book and reflect upon applications to your own practice. A glossary and list of further resources have been included, which will be of special interest to those readers enrolled in academic programs.

I commend *Coaching children: sports science essentials* to you as an excellent, user-friendly way to increase your knowledge, competence and personal confidence as a coach in children's sport today. The information should help you to become a better coach.

Coaches need to remain up-to-date with the latest sports science research and techniques. If we can take on board Kelly's recommendations and engage children in fun, motivating and meaningful programs, we can reduce the rates of attrition and instead reward children with enjoyment and fitness, enhancing the likelihood of lifelong participation in sport.

Janet L Currie
Senior Lecturer and Coordinator
Personal Development, Health and Physical Education
University of Technology, Sydney

CONTENTS

A NOTE FROM THE AUTHOR

As a coach or fitness professional, practical experience is usually what you draw upon when designing your exercise programs for children. Rightly so, as these types of roles are highly practical and there is no substitute for your real experience. But imagine if you were given an overview of relevant and practical sports science knowledge—would you feel more confident that you were designing the safest and most effective exercise programs for the children in your care?

This book contains suggestions for designing exercise programs to cater for children's physical and social development, as well as information on sports nutrition, sports psychology, injury management and much more. The technical sports science information has been distilled into a format that is practical and easy to read. As a coach or fitness professional, you should be able to read each chapter and learn a number of techniques you can apply immediately.

Discussion of children throughout the book is based on the ages of 8 to 15 years. It is between these ages that children usually start participating in organised sport, before they move towards senior and adult competition. This is also the age range where most of the research has been focused. To date, there are minimal sports sciences coaching references that concentrate on training children. This educational resource offers you a wide range of practical sports science information based on research, books and organisational documents.

This book took 18 months to research and write. I believe the time was well worth investing so that as a coach or fitness professional you have access to credible knowledge you can use out on the field to help children have a safe, effective and enjoyable time exercising.

Finally, I dedicate this book to Grant Perry, who encourages me to achieve my goals; to my sister, who is my essential support; and to Debbie Lee, one of the most positive and professional people you could meet.

Best of luck with your coaching.

Kelly Sumich

IMPROVING CHILDREN'S MOTOR SKILL DEVELOPMENT

Coaches play an important role in the development of a child's motor skills. Teaching basic skills such as running, throwing and catching provides a foundation for children to participate in future sporting activities and also contributes to the development of children's ongoing physical wellbeing. Understanding the motor skill development of a child and how to alter motor skill activity difficulty means you can set up an environment where children have the best chance of improvement.

This first chapter outlines:

▶ the classification of motor skills and how these can be tailored to suit a child's skill level
▶ three stages of motor skill learning, including how this information can be applied in a practical coaching setting
▶ the most effective way to structure training sessions to enhance motor skill development
▶ how to assess children's motor skill development.

CLASSIFICATION OF MOTOR SKILLS

Motor skills are voluntary, learnt movements made by the human body to achieve a task, such as a child twisting their body and moving their arm to throw a ball (Magill 2007).

Motor skills are classified into six categories: gross, fine, discrete, serial, closed and open. You can use knowledge about motor skill classification to tailor skill difficulty in training sessions. This is useful in setting tasks that match a child's ability and assist their developmental learning.

Gross and fine motor skills

The first classification of motor skills is related to the size of muscle groups used to perform an activity. When large muscle groups within the body create large action movements, such as during running, walking, swimming and jumping, these are termed gross motor skill movements. When a smaller number of muscles are used to create smaller action movements, such as writing and typing, these are classified as fine motor skills (Magill 2007).

Classifications of these skills are defined along a continuum, as some activities require both fine and gross motor skills in varying degrees. Golf is a good example of this. When a child performs a golf swing, they use their larger muscle groups, whereas putting involves smaller, more precise movements.

McFarland (2011) found that the time children spend indoors as opposed to outdoors playing has an impact on their motor skill development. Children spending more time indoors generally have higher levels of fine motor skills but lower levels of gross motor skill.

Davey (2012) highlighted the results of a recent study by the University of Sydney, which found that children's motor skill development is on the decline. Only 10 per cent of children in the research were able to master the four expected gross motor skills of a basic sprint run, a vertical jump, a side gallop and a leap by Year 2. The researcher Dr Louise Hardy was quoted in the article saying that 'parents mistakenly believe that children naturally learn these fundamental movement skills. But children need to be taught them'.

You may notice substantial differences in motor skill levels between today's child athletes compared to past groups. For you as a coach, depending on the motor skill levels of the children and their age, it may mean your training will need to focus or spend additional time on the development of gross motor skills. These can be incorporated using fun activities such as tunnel ball, dodging games, skipping, balance activities, obstacle courses, throwing and jumping games. The development of gross motor skills can be enhanced through activities specific to the sport you coach. For example, in netball, passing the ball is a common sport skill development activity, however, it is also beneficial in developing the gross motor skills of throwing and catching.

Major gross motor skills such as jumping, throwing and catching start to become more refined around the ages of 9 or 10. The gross motor skill of hitting, such as in softball, usually becomes more refined at a later age—around 14 years of age.

Discrete and serial motor skills

Motor skills can also be classified according to how they start and finish. If a skill has a definite start and finish it is called a discrete skill. Examples of discrete skills including hitting a baseball, a free throw in basketball or a free kick for goal in football. Some discrete skills can also be completed in a series. Bouncing a basketball and then catching it on the spot is a discrete skill; however, dribbling the basketball along the court is a serial motor skill (McMorris 2004).

When coaching a new motor skill, it is recommended that you introduce the discrete skill first before moving on to teaching the serial motor skills. If we use the previous basketball example, the child learns and achieves the discrete action of bouncing and catching first. Once the child seems comfortable with this skill they then move on to bouncing the basketball multiple times without stopping to catch it. As a coach, you can set challenges such as seeing how many times the child can bounce the ball without stopping, and then having them move while bouncing the ball (Magill 2007).

Closed and open motor skills

Closed and open motor skills are defined by the environment in which the skill is performed. A closed motor skill is an activity where the target or object is stationary and/or the environment is stable. This type of skill is deemed self-paced, because the child can normally choose when to perform the activity and is not influenced by external factors. Examples of closed motor skills include hitting the ball off a tee and a child swimming in their own training lane. In these activities there are minimal external influences on the child performing the activity. This type of activity can be easier than an open motor skill (Magill 2007).

An open motor skill is used when the target or object is in motion and/or the environment is changing. Team sports such as soccer, football, netball and basketball involve a great deal of change, including where the players are, the direction of the ball, the speed of the ball and competing against others.

For optimal motor skill development, it is helpful, where possible, to start children learning closed motor skills first. This allows them to focus on learning the skill without having to also take in information from a moving target or a changing environment. These additional factors can be introduced once the child has mastered the basics of the skill (McMorris 2004). Table 1.1 lists examples of how coaches can alter the difficulty of an activity by changing it from a closed to an open motor skill.

Table 1.1   Examples of closed and open motor skills

Sport	Activity	Closed skill	Open skill
Baseball	Hitting the ball	Hitting the ball off a tee	Hitting the ball thrown by a pitcher
Basketball	Dribbling the ball	Dribbling the ball up and down the court	Dribbling the ball up and down the court with an opponent trying to steal the ball
Cycling	Riding a bike	Cycling on an indoor stationary bike on an easy, stable resistance	Cycling outside with external factors such as traffic and hills

Table 1.1 (continued)

Sport	Activity	Closed skill	Open skill
Gymnastics	Somersaulting	Performing the somersault	Performing the somersault with an apparatus such as a ball or a ribbon

FITTS AND POSNER'S THREE-STAGE MODEL OF MOTOR SKILL LEARNING

Motor skill learning is a continuous process where a child moves from being unable to master the basics to becoming competent. While this is a dynamic process, sports scientists have found it easier to guide coaches and others by classifying motor skill learning into stages. Fitts and Posner (1967) proposed a three-stage model of skill learning. To enhance motor skill development it is recommended that you alter your teaching style and training plans according to which of these three stages a child seems to fall within.

The cognitive stage of motor skill learning

The first stage of motor skill development is where a child focuses on the thought processes of each movement. This means that when they are being taught how to complete a serve in tennis, the child will separate the information into individual components to recreate the movement. The child will go to perform the serve and will be thinking of how to hold the racquet, how to toss the ball in the air, when and how to pull the arm back and when and how to strike the ball. The cognitive stage is characterised by a large number of errors and a low consistency in performance (Rink 2002).

Application to coaching

When a child is in the initial stage of learning a new motor skill, it is recommended that you keep your description to the key elements. This will minimise the chance of causing confusion or information overload from the child having too many elements to think about. Feedback should be focused on the achievement of the key elements being taught rather than on performance outcome. For example, let the child know when they have completed a successful toss of the tennis ball in the air as opposed to measuring how many serves reach within the service box. It is likely that the child will experience a high number of errors and low performance output; focusing feedback on the key elements being taught can help maintain motivation regardless of performance levels.

In this stage of learning, children will not understand how to correct their own mistakes. This is because they lack the knowledge and experience of how the movement feels when correctly performed and because they cannot see their own performance to make a judgement. It is at this stage that your feedback is particularly important in helping a child understand what they did correctly and how to make improvements. It is also useful to keep the environment as neutral as possible by selecting mostly closed-skill tasks.

Children in this phase of learning have not yet established efficient methods of performing skills and thus will expend substantial amounts of energy. Initially, children are usually excited to perform a new skill but they can quickly tire. You will need to monitor energy levels to ensure children receive adequate rest.

The associative stage of motor skill learning

Transitioning into the second stage of motor skill learning is a dynamic process. The child will begin to think less about every element of the skill. They will also find they can start to tell when they feel they have performed the skill incorrectly and may even be able to fix the problem themselves. Fewer errors are made, consistency improves and the movements become more fluid. This can be a motivating time for children as improvements and performance outcomes can start to happen rapidly.

The transition to this stage can be dependent on many factors such as the amount of practice and the level of motor skill difficulty of the activity.

Application to coaching

As a child moves from the cognitive to the associative stage, their motivation can be higher as they make fewer errors and feel more competent. You can start incorporating goal- and performance-oriented tasks, along with allocating additional time to practise as the child becomes more efficient at the skill and expends less energy. To make tasks more difficult, you may be able to introduce more open skills activities such as adding a varied environment and/or moving objects. Refer to Table 1.1 for ideas.

Children can also be given more freedom to incorporate their unique style. Some children may change the structure of the movement slightly to suit them and if this works to produce the same or a better outcome this can be accepted and encouraged. The only time this can cause a problem is if it puts the child at a higher risk of injury; then you should correct the child and explain your reasons.

When children move closer to the third stage of motor skill learning, performance improvement can slow down. Here, again, motivational techniques are important. Providing new, interesting and challenging games and activities along with setting goals can guide children to further develop their skills and maintain adherence to the sport.

The autonomous stage of motor skill learning

The autonomous stage of learning is when a child has practised and experienced the motor skills in many different settings and environments over a long period of time. The child can perform the skill automatically with a high consistency and performance level. They are also proficient in adjusting their own performance as they have vast experience on how the motor skill should be successfully carried out. It usually takes around ten or more years to reach this stage. As a result, children do not normally reach this level until they are adolescents or adults (Rink 2002).

Application to coaching
You are still important at this level in offering motivation, support and feedback and by keeping up-to-date with the latest sporting knowledge and techniques to pass on to the athlete.

STRUCTURING TRAINING SESSIONS TO ENHANCE MOTOR SKILL DEVELOPMENT

When teaching motor skills to children there are different ways you can structure the training sessions to improve development. These include:

▶ specificity of practice
▶ variability of practice
▶ mass or distributed training sessions
▶ teaching whole or part motor skills
▶ simplification of practice.

Specificity of practice
Specificity of practice relates to the theory that a child should practise the exact skill they want to develop and improve at. For example, if you want a child to learn how to become a soccer player, then teaching soccer-related skills is obviously going to enhance their motor skill development in this area. However, Capranica and Millard-Stafford (2011) and Moesch et al. (2011) found that participating in a broad range of sports does not hinder children in reaching an elite level. For those athletes interested in pursuing elite participation—with the exception of those sports where peak performance occurs at a younger age, such as gymnastics—specialisation is not required until the mid-teens. The risks of early specialisation can include greater attrition rates (children leaving the sport) and adverse physical and emotional health outcomes (Baker, Cobley & Thomas 2009).

It is important that children learn the motor skills for the sport you are teaching, but they should be allowed to participate in a range of sports.

Intense specialisation can commence around the mid-teens (15 or 16 years of age, as per Balyi's Long-Term Athlete Development model, see p. 59), if children show the interest and aptitude necessary for a more serious commitment to one sport.

Variability of practice

Variability of practice involves developing training sessions that have changing elements within the same sport. This could include changing the difficulty of the skills, the terrain, the speed or the duration. For example, if you were a running coach you could:

▶ vary the speed and duration of the runs—have children complete a long, slow run of 8 minutes in one session and then fast intervals of 30 seconds with 1 minute rest in the next session
▶ vary the terrain such as incorporating hill training or beach running.

If you were a tennis coach you could ask children to return a forehand drive to different sections of the return court.

The advantages of changing the variables are to:

▶ add an element of interest
▶ increase the range of motor skill experience of the child
▶ increase the body's adaptability in preparation for open skill sports that involve many changing variables such as basketball, soccer, netball and hockey.

Variability of practice works along similar principles to the way open skill sports create more difficulty through their changing environment. As with an open skill, variability of practice will be dependent on what stage of motor skill learning the child is at and the difficulty of the sport. Adding too many variables for children in the first stages of motor skill learning may be overwhelming and can result in anxiety rather than motor skill development.

As a coach, you need to decide what motor skill level the children are at. If they are within the second associative stage of motor skill learning or higher, then you can think about variability of practice. If you coach children at the initial cognitive motor skill learning stage, then the children will have enough difficulty mastering the basics without the need for variability of practice.

Table 1.2   Examples of variability of practice

Sport	Variability of practice suggestions
Football	▶ Practise kicking goals from different distances and angles ▶ Add varying speed and agility games
Netball	▶ Swap the players' positions around ▶ Practise passing the ball with two netballs instead of one
Hockey	▶ Change the surface for training one day—move from grass to astroturf ▶ Introduce a new penalty corner strategy
Diving	▶ Change the height of the boards children dive from ▶ Ask children to perform a different dive. It does not have to be more difficult, just different
Tennis	▶ Mix the sessions up, focusing on serves one week and on volleys the next ▶ Ask children to return a forehand drive to different places on the return court
Rowing	▶ Add interval sessions of varying durations

Mass or distributed training sessions

A mass training session gives little rest time over one large block of training. This type of training is more suitable for adults, especially those with limited training time available. Training sessions incorporating rest periods are called distributed training sessions and this type of training can be of more benefit in improving children's motor skill development.

For a coach, the challenge is how to incorporate rest periods without children becoming bored or restless. Options can include:

- conducting regular drink breaks
- having one child exercising and another watching, giving feedback or counting
- having small groups of children lined up so that when one child is exercising, the others wait. If the group is small enough and the activity is brief enough this will keep the children from getting bored and provide them with appropriate rest periods.

Distributed training can also refer to a number of shorter sessions spread throughout the week. For example, conducting three training sessions of 1 hour rather than one mass training session of 3 hours' duration. The shorter, more frequent training sessions are preferable for motor skill development.

Teaching whole or part motor skills

Deciding whether to demonstrate the whole motor skill or break it down into parts can be complex. Basically, it is dependent on two aspects of the skill: the complexity and the organisation.

Complexity of the motor skill

The complexity of a motor skill relates to how many parts are involved. When teaching a motor skill with high complexity, you need to break the skill down into parts. A tennis serve has around 6 or 7 components and is considered highly complex. This means when teaching children how to perform a tennis serve, you need to show them what the skill looks like when all the parts are put together so they have an understanding of the end result, but explain each of the serve's individual components separately (Magill 2007).

Organisation of the motor skill

The second aspect to deciding whether to teach a motor skill as a whole or in parts is its organisation. This relates to the flow of the motor skill. For example, the jump shot in basketball has a level of high organisation. When a motor skill has high organisation, it is better to teach the whole skill. It can be very disruptive to the flow of the skill if it is taught in parts and it can be difficult for you to stop in mid–skill while demonstrating (Magill 2007).

A last consideration when deciding whether to teach children a motor skill in its entirety or broken into parts is the age of the child. Younger children may have difficulty learning the whole aspect of a skill, so skills with high organisation may need to be left until they grow older. Alternatively, they could be taught a simplified version of the skill.

Simplification of practice

Simplification of practice is about using techniques to make it easier for the child to perform the motor skill. If a child is finding a motor skill too difficult, you could make the skill more closed, such as reducing external or environmental cues. Another common method of simplification is to adjust the playing field, such as using a smaller soccer oval or a lower netball goal post, or adjusting the equipment such as using a tennis ball in softball. The aim with this training principle is to gradually move the sequencing of skill development from simple to complex.

An interesting simplification method to guide motor skill development in some children is music. The rhythmic nature of music can help children by creating an auditory pacing system. You may be able to incorporate this technique in some of your training activities.

MOTOR SKILL ASSESSMENT

Performance and learning

One way you can assess motor skill development is by measuring the observable outcomes of a child's performance, such as how many serves a child makes within the tennis service box. The problem with this sort of evaluation is that in the initial stages of motor skill development, the child will experience a high number of errors and a high level of performance inconsistency. It can be more practical and confidence-building for children within this stage for you to limit your evaluation to observing motor skill learning and development.

General characteristics of skill learning

There are three general characteristics you can observe to evaluate a child's motor skill progress. These include:

▶ the child's level of improvement. When a child becomes more competent at performing a skill, they are noticeably better at it than when it was first attempted

▶ the child's level of consistency. When a child becomes more proficient at a motor skill they can competently perform the skill more often, for example, being able to keep the hockey ball from the opponents or marking the football without dropping it on most occasions.

▶ the child's level of adaptability. When a child becomes highly proficient at a motor skill they can perform the skill at this standard regardless of the changing internal (e.g. stress) and external (e.g. crowd) factors. For example, rhythmic gymnasts practise their routines so often they can perform them in front of large crowds with little change in performance outcomes. Their performance becomes automatic. Softball batters are deemed proficient if, regardless of the pitcher, they can sustain a certain batting average over the season.

Quantitative and qualitative assessment

Quantitative assessment involves assessing a child using statistical measurement, such as how quickly they can run 50 metres. The results can be compared to those of peers or can show improvements in the same child's performance over time.

A weakness of quantitative assessment is that it does not recognise why a child may be excelling or lagging behind their peers. A qualitative assessment is more observational and descriptive, and includes a greater range of factors presenting the reasons why. A qualitative assessment of a child running 50 metres might be, 'The child is very short for her age and has trouble matching stride length with her peers. The child, however, demonstrates an efficient running style'.

Summative assessment

Summative assessment is carried out at particular periods of time; for example, conducting a fitness test or a skill-based assessment every four weeks over three months. The aim is to monitor improvement over a set period of time, particularly when new training elements are added. This also offers you feedback on the effectiveness of your training program.

It is your responsibility to ensure that you are monitoring children's motor skill development, whether formally or informally, but children should have fun and enjoy their sport. A balance between monitoring, measurement and maintaining an enjoyable sporting environment is a challenge for coaches.

Identifying talented children

The identification of children with potential talent has been evolving and changing rapidly over time. Previously, talent identification included:

- measuring a body's dimensions (anthropometric testing)
- applying tests to measure skills and performance
- using experienced staff in observing and selecting potentially talented children.

The problem that has been identified with these methods is they do not consider barriers that prevent some talented children from going on to become elite athletes. Such barriers can include financial difficulties, lack of parental support, remote locations and psychological challenges such as anger or anxiety issues.

Talent identification programs are now researching and identifying a range of attributes and barriers a child may encounter during their training, competition and external lives that may prevent them from reaching their full potential. These additional factors can then be combined with body dimension measurements, skill and performance testing and observation to assist in evaluating a child's potential. The knowledge about potential barriers will also contribute to guiding coaches and carers on strategies to retain talented children in sport.

Talent identification can be problematic in accurately predicting athletic success, as many sports do not involve physical skill alone. Crespo and McInerney (2006) explain that in tennis, for example, there is also a substantial reliance on:

▶ decision-making processes
▶ mental strength to endure long-term rigorous training and to sustain concentration during long matches
▶ an ability to remain calm and focused under pressure.

A study by Vrljic and Mallet (2008) found that football talent identification coaches nominated speed, ball control and the desire to succeed as distinguishing talented players from those considered less talented.

Evaluating mental abilities is more difficult than assessing than physical skills, however, these still play an important role in talent identification. This is why both quantitative (statistical) and qualitative (descriptive, observation-based) methods of research and data collection can be useful in identifying talent.

A further challenge with talent identification in children is that they grow and develop at different rates. Those children excelling early on may be excelling due to being taller, stronger and more mature than their peers. The less mature children should not be discounted from future opportunities (Bailey, Morley & Dismore 2009). Offering talent identification on a yearly basis could help motivate children to continue motor skill development while they wait for their physical development to align with that of their peers.

Other external factors such as parental support, injuries and access to coaches, equipment and facilities can affect the rate of and opportunities for development of children. If, as a coach, you are considering offering a talent identification program to your athletes, you might want to think about the following factors.

▶ What criteria you are going to use for selection?
▶ Who makes the decisions?
▶ How is the talent identification program going to be funded?
▶ Who will design the program?
▶ How often will the talent identification occur?
▶ How will the additional training fit in with the need to avoid specialisation too early and the management of injuries occurring through overtraining?
▶ How will the management of the children who miss out be handled, including maintaining motivation, feelings of competence and enjoyment?
▶ Is there a minimum age and a target number for the group?
▶ Should you contact your national sporting organisation or a similar organisation for advice?

SUMMARY

▶ Motor skill development is essential in providing the basic foundations for children to perform in sport.
▶ Motor skills have classifications such as gross, fine, open, closed, discrete and serial.
▶ You can develop gross motor skills in children by incorporating activities such as tunnel ball, dodging games, skipping, balance activities, obstacle courses, throwing and jumping games.
▶ Altering motor skills from closed to open environments is an effective way to progress children's motor skill development.
▶ Fitts and Posner's three-stage model of motor skill learning is used to explain how you can adapt your teaching methods to enhance the learning and motor skill development of children.

▶ When children are learning new motor skills their performance and consistency will be low. The focus should be on learning the skill rather than measuring performance.

▶ You can structure training sessions to enhance children's motor skill development, including adding variability to the training sessions and selecting the most effective ways to teach motor skills by demonstrating either the whole or part of the motor skill.

REFLECTIVE QUESTIONS FOR THE COACH

⬙ How would you rate the level of gross motor skills in the children you coach? Does this mean you need to add more gross motor skill activities?

⬙ Are the children you coach able to cope with open motor skills? Do you have a list of skills you teach that could be made easier or more difficult through changing the skills from closed to open or moving from open to closed environments?

⬙ What stage in the Fitts and Posner's model do most of the children you coach fit into? What teaching strategies are recommended for this stage? Can you incorporate these into your coaching?

⬙ Are there any ways you could structure your training sessions differently to enhance motor skill development?

⬙ How detailed do you think the assessment of the children you coach should be? Which quantitative (statistical measurement) or qualitative (descriptive, observational) techniques would suit your sport and the age of the children you coach? Do you feel you need to assess the children?

⬙ Does your sport have talent identification? Do you think it is effective?

TAILORING CHILDREN'S EXERCISE TO CATER FOR THEIR PHYSICAL AND SOCIAL DEVELOPMENT

Understanding a child's physical and social development can help you tailor your training programs to be safe and effective. A child's body is significantly different to an adult's and their training programs need to be modified to accommodate these differences.

You also need to set your expectations and training challenges around a child's performance capabilities. What a child can achieve may be limited until they reach full physical, social and psychological development. Tailoring a child's training to an achievable level and respecting their limitations will help maintain their interest and progression in sport.

This chapter outlines:

- designing a training program to promote healthy physical growth in children
- the aerobic and anaerobic training capacity of children compared to adults
- children's social and emotional development and how you can nurture this development through sport
- practical training guidelines to cater for children's physical and social development in sport.

CHILDREN'S PHYSICAL DEVELOPMENT

Healthy bone growth

Children's bones do not fully fuse until their late teens or early twenties. This creates some concern about whether exercise will affect a child's bone growth and whether children are at higher risk of injury.

Instead of fully fused bones, children have a growth plate at either end of their long bones. This growth plate is made up of growing tissue as opposed to strong solid bones and the softness of the growth plate can place children at risk of injury. Adults tend to sustain ligament injuries, because of the weakness of the ligaments compared to the strength of their fully fused bones (American Academy of Orthopaedic Surgeons 2010; Gerrard 1993).

Children performing in sports that involve collisions, such as football and hockey, are at greater risk of sustaining bone growth injuries, as are participants in sports with repetitive physical loading, such as gymnastics, distance running and baseball. If children sustain or are suspected to sustain a bone injury it is important they see a doctor. If bone growth injuries are not treated properly, the bone may be prone to curvature or result in growth that is unequal in length to normal bone growth. Boys are more likely to sustain growth plate injuries than girls as their growth plates usually fuse at a later age.

According to a study by Caine, DiFiori and Maffuli (2006), most growth plate injuries are sustained by children aged between 13 and 17 years and recovery outcomes are generally positive with no long-term damage.

Exercise that is weight-bearing has a positive impact on a child's bone development. Weight-bearing exercise involves children carrying their own body weight, such as when running or doing a push-up. If a child is involved in a non-weight-bearing sport, such as swimming, it is recommended for bone development that they also participate in weight-bearing exercise throughout the week and consume the recommended calcium intake.

Boreham and McKay's (2011) research findings support the concept that moderate to vigorous physical activity, such as team sports training, and short bouts of high-impact activity, such as jumping activities, promote bone growth in children. But repetitious, high-impact activities should not be included with great frequency and continuously throughout the year. Repetitious high-impact activities are those that place a medium to high level of strain on a particular part of the body. For example, long-distance running can place a strain on the shin bones; playing netball most days of the week can place strain on the knees; the constant throwing action in tee ball can place strain on the shoulder.

The fundamental message is that exercise is positive for children as it contributes to healthy bone growth, but high-intensity, repetitious exercise needs to be avoided as this increases a child's risk of bone fracture and injury (Gerrard 1993). Children should not be completing the same activities over and over again on a daily basis. You can minimise the risk of growth plate injury by:

▶ varying training intensities by providing low, moderate and vigorous sessions
▶ ensuring training sessions have a variety of activities that use different muscles and body parts.

Gymnastics coaches can move children from floor activities, which have high body impact on the lower legs, to allowing children to land in the foam pit while learning a new skill, to the parallel bars. It is about adding a variety of skills and muscle use exercises to the training program.

Calcium is one of the essential nutrients children need to consume to contribute to healthy bone growth. Information on the recommended calcium intake and the best times for children to consume calcium for sport are outlined in Chapter 6.

Healthy muscle development

As children grow older, they steadily develop muscle strength and growth. When boys reach puberty, muscle development starts to rapidly increase with their level of testosterone. Muscle mass will make up around 45 per cent of their body weight, which generally contributes to them being broader in the shoulders and having a higher metabolism, prompting them to eat more. Girls show a steadier increase in muscle mass peaking at around 30 to 35 per cent of their body weight.

The use of weight training as a method to develop muscle strength in children is debated; however, the Australian Strength and Conditioning Association (2007), the Australian Sports Commission (n.d. b) and Sibte (2003) all support the use of weight training for children if:

▶ a properly qualified strength and conditioning coach designs and/ or teaches the sessions
▶ the child is over the age of 8
▶ only low weights are used, for example 1- to 3-kilogram dumbbells
▶ proper technique is taught and continually monitored
▶ repetitions and volume are very low, such as 8 to 15 repetitions repeated twice
▶ non-explosive weight techniques are employed, i.e. avoid dead lifts and clean and jerk lifts until the child is more experienced with weight training
▶ the exercises are kept simple (lunges and squats holding weights; shoulder presses using weights) so that basic techniques can be learnt (Beihoff & Pop 2009; Faigenbaum et al. 2009).

Prior to puberty, girls and boys do not develop significant muscle bulk from weight training. Children experience increases in strength from improved muscle coordination and motor unit activation, which contribute to a more efficient signal being sent to the muscle, creating movement and improving strength (Granacher et al. 2011). Once puberty is reached, boys may start to notice increased muscle bulk, which in turn can create increased muscle power and strength beyond that of girls.

While older children can participate in weight training, they can also access other types of training to improve strength. You can give children exercises where they are using their own body weight such as in push-ups, handstands, cartwheels, sit-ups and the plank. Children can also participate in plyometric exercises such as jumping over low obstacles, skipping and bounding. These are all effective strength and conditioning training methods (Beihoff & Pop 2009; Johnson, Salzberg & Stevenson 2011). More information about these techniques is presented in Chapter 3.

Before children reach the age of 12, both boys and girls generally have the same muscle mass and strength. After this time, if you train both sexes together, then you will need to be mindful of the growing strength differences. These strength differences can also start to vary between boys of the same age.

Nervous system

The nervous system is a series of nerve fibres that conducts impulses from the brain to different parts of the body and back again. During exercise, the effective transmission of these impulses contributes to reaction time, skilled movement, balance, agility and coordination. The nervous system does not fully develop until after puberty, so while you can improve a child's reaction times and agility through training, they may still have limited performance ability until their nervous system becomes fully developed.

Cardiovascular and lung function

A child's heart and lungs are smaller than an adult's so their body's ability to pump blood and oxygen from their lungs is lower. By late puberty, children reach a similar blood and oxygen output from the heart and lungs as adults. Children's lung size and function also reaches full capacity at this time.

Body composition

Children have the same needs as adults to balance its food and fluid intake against their exercise and resting metabolic output in order to maintain a healthy body weight. However, if children exercise at the same intensity as adults, they exert a higher metabolic rate.

The World Health Organization (2010) stated its concern about the physical inactivity of children and the current and growing rate of childhood obesity. This trend is also found in Australia, with one quarter of Australian children (or around 600000 children aged from 5 to 17 years) in 2007–08 being classified as overweight or obese. This is up four percentage points from 1995 (Australian Bureau of Statistics 2011).

Obese children are four times more likely than children of a healthy weight to become overweight when they are adults. Your responsibilities involve not only focusing on developing children's motor skills and fitness but also enhancing their self-esteem and love of exercise. If children feel good about exercising they are more likely to participate in exercise later in life.

During puberty, girls can start to put on weight and experience a widening of the hips. This may create stress and feelings of self-consciousness about their bodies and reduce participation in exercise. The Australian Sports Commission (n.d. a) reports that girls 'start to drop out of sport at an alarming rate when they are in the 12 to 14 year age group' and 'a poor self-image at a delicate stage of a girl's transition into adulthood is the main reason causing young girls to abandon their sporting activities'. It is important as a coach that you encourage girls to continue exercising as this in itself can assist in maintaining a healthy body weight. Girls at this stage may need specialised supportive sports bras and good information about their nutritional needs, such as their need to have an adequate intake of iron. Encouraging the social aspect of sport, such as offering more team games and social events, can also help.

Thermal stress

Children suffer more than adults in extremely hot temperatures. They do not have the same ability as adults to dissipate heat. It is not until they reach puberty that a child's sweat mechanisms to cool their body become as efficient as an adult's. Children also suffer greater heat loss than adults during colder temperatures (Burke & Deakin 2008; Sports Medicine Australia 2008).

As a coach it is important for you to have strategies in place during extreme temperatures. In summer, hold training during the cooler part of the day, allow children to stop and drink water, exercise in the shade if possible and shorten the session if need be. On colder days, do not let children stand around for long periods of time in minimal clothing. Allow them to keep their jumpers and tracksuit pants on during the warm-up and, if they take them off during the training session, remind them to put them back on during the cool-down.

AEROBIC AND ANAEROBIC TRAINING CAPACITY IN CHILDREN

Aerobic training capacity

Aerobic training is exercise conducted at levels that children can sustain for long periods of time, such as walking and slow jogging. Throughout aerobic exercise, children have enough oxygen to perform the activity and usually feel comfortable. There are different training methods that can be applied to develop a child's aerobic ability. These include:

▶ intermittent exercise such as running 200 to 600 metres, or repeating a sporting activity which lasts around 1 to 3 minutes followed by a period of rest
▶ long, slow, continuous exercise such as runs or activities for a duration of about 10 minutes.

It is a good idea to mix both styles of aerobic training to avoid boredom. Children are generally suited to, and have a preference for, intermittent training (Rowland 2002). If coaching children under the age of 10, long, continuous exercise should ideally be for no more than 10 minutes before allowing children a rest period.

Anaerobic training capacity

Anaerobic training is exercise that exceeds the body's ability to transport blood and oxygen to the heart and working muscles. If the required oxygen needs are not met due to exercising at such a high intensity then lactic acid is produced as a by-product. High rates of lactic acid result in the body needing to slow down or stop. This can occur after 2 minutes of high-intensity exercise.

For very short intensity exercise, such as the golf swing or a 50-metre sprint, the body has around 10 seconds of energy stored in the muscles, and will not produce lactic acid even if oxygen supplies are low. This store of chemical energy is called the adenosine triphosphate (ATP) system. If exercise is continued at high intensity after the ATP stores are depleted and oxygen needs are not met, then the body will move into anaerobic exercise.

In 2003, a sports scientist named Tim Noakes suggested that the fatigue caused during intense anaerobic exercise actually resulted from the brain sending signals to create muscle fibre contraction reduction to protect the body from irreversable damage. He claimed that short anaerobic training sessions can be a method of training the brain to run the body at high intensity and accept that it can do so at increasingly higher intensities without causing damage. Anaerobic training can increase fitness quickly, however, if performed too often and for too long it can cause overtraining and a higher risk of injury.

Children have a significantly lower anaerobic training capacity compared to that of adults (Cross & Lyle 1999; Rowland 2002). As a rough guide, a child aged around 11 years can manage about one-third of the training load of an adult. If the child is a runner, they should not exceed a total of 8 to 10 kilometres in one training session. This includes all the accumulated distance in that one session, such as during the warm-up, the main component and the cool-down.

From 15 years of age, some children can manage a training program closer to an adult level. After this age children can start to cope with more intense competition, however, they may not be able to sustain a peak level of training for as long as an adult can. Children at this age should not be trained with regular high-intensity training sessions for more than six or seven weeks at a time. You can plan training to help older children reach peak fitness without injury by structuring their six to seven weeks of intense, highly focused training just prior to a major competition. If there are multiple important competitions throughout the year, older children should be scheduled with no more than three peaks. Always ensure children receive sufficient rest for recovery.

CHILDREN'S SOCIAL AND EMOTIONAL DEVELOPMENT

The age of a child can affect the way in which they respond to coaching instructions. For example, a child under the age of 15 years may not be socially developed enough to separate judgements about their physical ability from those about their worth as a person. The following subsections explain how you can use information about the way that a child develops socially and emotionally to enhance their sporting ability and self-esteem.

Children's attention span

Children under the age of 8 have a very short attention span. At this age, children are super-energetic and enjoy a variety of activities including climbing, jumping, running and hopping, however, they tire quickly and need lots of rest breaks. They also tire around early afternoon. Activities for children under the age of 8 should be based around play that is highly energetic and varied with lots of rest opportunities. Instructions should be kept to a bare minimum (Humphrey 2003).

From the age of 9, children can be introduced to more organised games. These children have a slightly longer attention span to listen to more than the most basic of instructions. While children at 9 display an amazing amount of energy, their aerobic training ability, particularly for continuous exercise, is still low. Children at this age can play for hours if the exercise is intermittent and includes lots of variety.

Around the age of 10, children become more interested in developing and learning skills. They will be more inclined to listen to instructions and enjoy activities that focus on skill development rather than being solely or mainly play-oriented. The fun and play aspect should, however, still be largely present (Australian Sports Commission 2008).

Gradually, from the age of 10, children will gain a greater ability to focus and listen to your instructions and will be able to engage in more activities structured towards skill development.

Peer approval

Around the age of 9, children start to recognise, seek approval and be influenced by their peers. This may mean children start to become distracted by others within the group. If this occurs, you can start to develop more challenging activities to help keep children occupied.

By the age of 11, some children are starting to develop physically, earlier than their peers. This can cause feelings of self-consciousness. In some cases, their bodies develop so quickly that they can become uncoordinated and clumsy, which can be distressing for some children. Positive feedback and tailoring exercise for different ability levels can help children move through this stage more confidently, more successfully and with less chance of feeling ostracised.

Once children reach the age of 11 they usually develop a strong team spirit and they really enjoy the social companionship exercise can offer. You can nurture this development through incorporating more group and teamwork activities.

There can also be a lot of silliness with girls and boys around the age of 11 and onwards. These factors cannot really be eliminated; it is the nature of their age. As a coach, it is best to accept this. On most occasions, keeping the children busy with varied exercise activities will keep them on task.

Competitiveness

An understanding of sporting competition is not normally reached until after the age of 9. After this time and by the age of 12, most children become mature enough to participate in competitive sports with appropriate supervision (Patel, Pratt & Greydanus 2002). As children move from play into sport, they will start to notice their skills and abilities in comparison with those of other children. While a child can compete, it is important that you teach them to focus on their own performance rather than compare themselves with others. This motto can be incorporated in training, for example, timing children for a set performance and then timing them again at a later date. The aim is to compare their own times and not assess themselves against other children. Most children will improve over time so this is a positive method of encouraging a child's development and self-esteem; not every child will be able to win, but every child can improve on their own performance. You should still incorporate many activities in your training that are play-like, where there is minimal comparison, particularly for younger children.

It is important to remember that children will likely not have the coping strategies and abilities of adults. Refer to Chapter 5 to find out more about how you can assist children to manage the stress of competition.

As children become older, their competitiveness, as with adults, will vary dramatically. On the whole, boys are generally more competitive than girls, though this is not an absolute. It is important that you accept and support boys who are not competitive in nature and also girls who are.

You may also need to start tailoring your feedback and motivational tactics to match children's differing reactions to competition. Some children excel from the excitement and challenge of competition whereas other children need far more support and encouragement.

All children need positive reinforcement, tasks set at a level they can achieve and an enjoyable learning environment.

Children can feel less competition anxiety if they are involved in a team sport rather than an individual sport. It may help to arrange their game and skill activities in groups.

Social comparison

Children want to please their carers and the adults in their lives. Children become attuned to whether you, as a coach, are happy with them, why and when. They also become aware of the attention being directed to other children in the group. Being conscious of this can be important.

From the age of 9, children become more conformist in attitude, wanting to be like each other and not stand out. While children like individual feedback, it helps if corrective feedback is given discreetly.

From the age of 10, children start to become more self-conscious of their bodies. This is particularly true for girls and may affect their participation. Strategies to deal with this are explained on page 23.

From the age of 11, children begin working on their social identity. One method of developing this is through comparing their values and opinions with those of other children, mainly of the same sex. The social aspect of exercise can be a healthy way for children to socialise and develop a positive connection with exercise and with their friends.

Group play

Children really enjoy play, especially with other children. They enjoy testing, using and developing their skills.

Humphrey (2003) found that children around the ages of 5 and 6 work best in small groups. Children of this age are self-centred, like to be first in games and are indifferent to whether the children in the group are of a different sex. At this age they also appreciate a great deal of praise.

From the age of 7, children start to want individual recognition for their achievements. Children of this age are not always good losers though they can start to show greater signs of cooperation in groups. You may be able to manage children that demonstrate unhappiness at losing by evaluating the difficulty of the task and the pressure on the child to win. You may also be able to:

▶ modify a child's expectations and remind them of the many improvements they have made so far

▶ explain to them (if they are in the older age group) about skill development and how the initial phase is characterised by a lower performance output and consistency, but that this will improve

▶ avoiding scoring or measuring performance during training sessions for a period of time. Refocus if need be on training sessions that emphasise fun and play.

From the age of 8, children start to gather in and form groups that are made up of the same sex. Children at this age also start to experience longer periods of cooperative play.

You can start incorporating more individual tasks and challenging activities with children aged 9. This is also when children may start to show more interest in participating in sporting activities outside school, particularly those shared with friends.

Substantial group work activities and the opportunity to socialise can be positive inclusions offered at training. Social interaction can become one of the main reasons children (and then later, adults) find exercise so enjoyable and motivating.

Emotions

Children can be very emotional. These emotions are usually released at high intensity, though normally do not last long. Distraction tactics can sometimes work, especially as children's emotions are subject to rapid change. The challenge, though, is that every child can react differently to similar circumstances and some react badly to gain attention. It is important not to use fear tactics or to use exercise as a punishment.

Humphrey (2003) found that children's three greatest fears with participating in sport were getting hurt, losing and not playing well. As a coach, you can help create a positive training environment by:

- teaching children to focus on their own improvements rather than comparing themselves against other children
- providing lots of praise and encouragement
- providing opportunities for equal participant time—do not leave a child weaker in skill or fitness level on the bench
- placing children in the appropriate sporting team level
- allowing children to make mistakes
- attempting to provide for individual differences in skill level and personality
- emphasising group activity outcomes as well as individual outcomes.

Appealing to 'the future' does not normally work with younger children. Children have not yet developed the intellectual capability to analyse current events and their impact on future outcomes, so, unlike adults, they do not worry about the future.

PRACTICAL TRAINING GUIDELINES TO CATER FOR CHILDREN'S PHYSICAL AND SOCIAL DEVELOPMENT

Equal training and game time

You should ensure that each child receives an equal opportunity to participate in developing their skills and fitness. Children need time to practise. This is not going to happen if they spend most of their time on the sidelines. If children who develop later than their peers are not offered the opportunity to fully develop their skills, this could prevent them from reaching their potential once they are grown.

Hill and Green (2008) explain that having fewer players in a smaller area of play improves participation and allows children more game-play experience. Their increased involvement contributes to increased player satisfaction, enjoyment and adherence to the sport. Hill and Green also recommend minimising the use of substitute players, so children can participate in the full game where possible.

Modified training and game play

Depending on the age of the children, a modified game may need to be incorporated to cater for fitness and skill levels. This can be achieved through altering the size of the field, reducing game time, changing the motor skill level or altering the rules of the activity. The Australian Sports Commission or your sport's national coaching organisation may also be able to give you further advice on suitable ways to modify training and game play.

Tailoring training for healthy bone development

You should ensure that you design training programs that involve a varying level of intensity, activities that incorporate a variety of muscle groups and provision of adequate rest. This will avoid creating stress and strain on growing bones, through minimising repetitious high-intensity activities.

Catering for different physical abilities

Around the age of 12 (or sometimes earlier) children can start to physically develop at vastly different rates. You can cater for this by matching children with similar levels of physical development, especially for activities reliant on physical size, strength and ability.

Nutrition

Coaches can teach children and carers about the basics of nutrition, such as the recommended calcium intake for healthy bone development. These details are outlined in Chapter 6.

Strength and conditioning

Strength and conditioning training options can be incorporated into a child's training program to enhance their physical development. These can include plyometric exercises, weight training and using a child's own body weight. Sports Medicine Australia (2008, p. 11) recommends that 'a strength training program should increase gradually and focus on correct technique'. The program should also be properly supervised and maximal lifts avoided until children reach full physical and skeletal maturity. Refer to Chapter 3 (pp. 48–9) for more information on these types of training.

Thermal stress

Children can be kept cooler during hotter weather by allowing drink stops, training in the shade and where possible training during the coolest parts of the day. When the weather is cold, encourage children to keep their jumpers and tracksuits on during the warm-up and cool-down and ensure they do not stand around for long periods of time getting cold.

Children involved in water sport activities or those who are subject to wet weather conditions will experience increased heat loss. Carers should ensure their children have spare warm clothes in these conditions (Sports Medicine Australia 2008).

Aerobic and anaerobic training

You should plan to incorporate a mixture of aerobic and anaerobic exercise in children's training. The volume of each will depend on the type of sport you coach. If you coach swimming, then the training normally incorporates more aerobic-based activities, whereas team sports such as netball and football will have more of a mixture of the two types of training.

Ratel et al. (2004) found that giving children 10 intervals of 10 seconds at just above maximal aerobic speed (so around 8 to 9 out of 10 work effort) during their training session increased their aerobic and anaerobic fitness levels. Children also recovered quicker from these higher-intensity intervals than adults. So while children have lower aerobic and anaerobic training capacities than adults, they suit short, high-intensity intermittent exercise. You can combine this type of training with skill development and game play.

SUMMARY

▶ Children's bones are not fully fused until their late teenage years or early twenties. Instead, children have a growth plate at the ends of their long skeletal bones, made up of growing tissue as opposed to solid bone.

▶ You need to avoid repetitious, high-impact training, which risks injury of the growth plate. In extreme cases, this can lead to curvature of the bone and uneven bone growth. If children are involved in high-impact training then a variety of training exercises and muscle group focus can significantly reduce the risk.

▶ Exercise, particularly weight-bearing exercise, contributes to enhanced healthy bone growth in children.

▶ Plyometric exercises, weight training (under recommended guidelines) and use of children's own body weight for resistance can contribute to healthy muscle growth and development.

▶ Children's nervous systems, cardiovascular systems and lung function are all developing during childhood and can influence performance by reducing their aerobic and anaerobic capacity.

▶ Childhood obesity is a growing concern. You can assist in reducing childhood obesity through not only focusing on developing children's motor skills and fitness levels but through enhancing their self-esteem and enjoyment of exercise.

▶ Children suffer more in extreme temperatures than adults do, and you will need to have measures in place to cater for this.

▶ Children have a reduced aerobic and anaerobic capacity compared to adults. Children are more suited to intermittent training rather than long, continuous training.

▶ Support comparison of children's performance against themselves rather than other children before the age of 15 years, as they may not be socially developed enough to separate judgements about their physical ability from those about their worth as people.

▶ From around the age of 11 children develop a strong team spirit and enjoy the social companionship exercise can offer. You can nurture this development through incorporating more group and teamwork activities.

REFLECTIVE QUESTIONS FOR THE COACH

◈ Is the sport you coach high in intensity and repetitious in the activities children are completing? Can you incorporate ways to alter the intensity and vary the muscle groups involved?

◈ In the sport you coach, do you need to group children of similar physical development together for safety? Is there a mixture of children and adults that you train?

◈ Do you have a plan to develop children's strength?

◈ Do you think it is your role to teach carers and children about nutrition?

◈ Is the sport you coach more aerobic or anaerobic in nature? What activities do you set to develop children's aerobic and anaerobic fitness? What levels of aerobic and anaerobic activities should you avoid for the sport you coach?

◈ What age group are you coaching and what level of attention span do the children have?

◈ Do you need lots of activities with few instructions or do you coach older children interested in more detailed instruction? How do you incorporate rest periods for children without them becoming bored?

◈ Is your sport a team sport? What amount of group work do you think you need to include? Are you using group work effectively to create rest? Do you have ways to encourage team spirit?

- Are the children you coach involved in competition? What focus on competitiveness do you place in training? At what age do you think children should become competitive? Do you have a preference on how you guide children in managing the competitiveness of sport? Do the children you coach need varied motivational tactics because of their reaction to competition?

- What do you think is the appropriate amount of positive feedback for the group you coach? Is it necessary for you to formally monitor the children's ability and progress? Would you say this has a positive or negative impact on children's development and enjoyment of the sport?

- Do you need to set tasks with varying difficulty levels because the children you coach have substantially different fitness and skill levels? Are the children you coach given equal practice and competition time?

DESIGNING EFFECTIVE TRAINING PROGRAMS

Coaches are responsible for designing and conducting children's training sessions. Most coaches have participated in the sport they are coaching and bring a wealth of knowledge and possibly coaching qualifications they can draw upon.

This chapter aims to assist you in identifying scientific training principles to develop effective training programs for the children you coach. Elements of this information should be useful to combine with your own knowledge and experiences.

The training principles explained in this chapter include:

- elements to consider when designing a training program for children
- basic principles of designing a training program
- physical components to incorporate in a training program
- methods to improve training adherence.

ELEMENTS TO CONSIDER WHEN DESIGNING A TRAINING PROGRAM FOR CHILDREN

There are four basic elements to consider when designing a training program for children. These elements consist of frequency, duration, intensity and mode of exercise.

Frequency

Frequency relates to how often a child trains per day and per week, and can depend on many factors including how old the child is, how expensive the training is, what carers can afford, the ability of carers to drop the child at training and whether the child is participating in a range of other sports and exercise activities. The main principle to consider is, the higher the frequency of training, the lower the intensity or duration of training should be. This is to prevent the child from overtraining and potentially sustaining an injury or becoming excessively tired (Heyward 2010).

The National Physical Activity Guidelines for Australian children aged from 5 to 18 years is 60 minutes of moderate to vigorous activity per day (Department of Health and Ageing 2004a, 2004b). Children have a great deal of energy and an ability to train daily, however, frequency needs to be balanced with intensity and duration of training. As a coach, it is a good idea to understand what other sporting activities and exercise a child does throughout the week.

It is also important to consider the level of skill involved in the sport. If the skill level in the sport is high, as with golf or tennis, then the child will need to practise more frequently. Children in the first cognitive stage of motor skill learning will tire quickly as they are not yet efficient at performing the skill. This means duration may need to be shortened or more rest periods included.

Duration

Duration relates to the length of time of each training session. Duration should be shorter for higher-intensity and frequent training unless a great deal of rest time is included in the session.

For children aged between 6 and 15 years, training duration should be equal to or less than 1 hour. However, as mentioned, you can change this to fit in with how frequently the child is exercising, the intensity of training, the rest periods offered during the training session and the child's training goals. Sometimes when a child is closer to adolescence they may be competing seriously and training seven days a week, with some sessions lasting a few hours. These children are normally performing intermittent exercises, which are stop–start related exercise, and taking rest periods throughout the training session (Heyward 2010).

Intensity

Intensity relates to the level of exertion during exercise. The general rule is that with higher-intensity exercise, the training frequency and duration should decrease. Research by Ratel, Duche and Williams (2006) found that children prefer intermittent exercise that involves medium- to high-intensity training for a short duration, followed by a rest. This process is then repeated. High-intensity activities are also useful in contributing to reducing the risk of obesity and increasing cardiovascular fitness in children. As mentioned, though, remember that high-intensity exercise must be planned with consideration of rest, duration and frequency to assist in avoiding injuries and overtraining.

Symptoms of overtraining

If children have reached the point of overtraining, or are close to it, they may exhibit:

▶ a reduction in motivation
▶ persistent fatigue and reduced performance
▶ ongoing muscle soreness
▶ more colds due to a lowered immune system
▶ increased sensitivity to problems including crying, anger and irritable behaviour (Noakes 2003).

If you find that one of the children you are coaching shows some or all of these symptoms, ask the child what exercise activities they have been doing in addition to your training. The child may need to rest to recover from overtraining and then change their training to a more manageable level. Discussion will need to take place with the child's carer.

Mode of exercise

Mode of exercise is the type of sport the child is participating in and relates to the goals and objectives of a child's training program. It is a similar concept to specificity of practice, which is explained on page 8. If the child's goal is to learn how to play tennis, then most, if not all, of the training activities you present should be centred on learning tennis skills and the fitness needs of this sport.

Cross training is sometimes introduced to add interest and avoid injuries. Cross training is when a child trains in a different activity or sport to the one related to their goal. A tennis coach can design a circuit class to complement the tennis training or have children participate in a beach running session, for instance. This class will not necessarily increase their tennis skills but will aid overall fitness and add variety.

For most children, the aim of exercising in the early years is to expose them to a wide variety of activities in a fun environment. They do not need to specialise until their mid-teenage years if they are interested in pursuing national or elite competition (Australian Sports Commission 2008).

BASIC PRINCIPLES OF TRAINING DESIGN

As a coach, there are a number of basic principles to consider when designing a training program for children. These are:

- specificity
- progressive overload
- training periodisation
- individual variability
- diminishing returns
- reversibility
- age.

Specificity

Specificity was discussed in the first chapter. This concept involves designing training that directly relates to the child's exercise goal, so if you are coaching basketball, your training will be centred on basketball activities and games.

With the exception of gymnastics, ballet, swimming and in some cases tennis, it is recommended that children experience a wide range of sports and activities rather than specialising too early. This will allow children to develop a wide range of key motor skills and discover an interest in one or more sports. As mentioned, children do not need to specialise until the mid-teenage years if they wish to pursue national or elite competition, except for those sports that involve elite competition at a very early age.

Progressive overload

If a person does the same exercise at the same frequency, intensity and duration for a long period of time, the body adapts and improvements will no longer occur. Progressive overload avoids this stagnation. It is important to offer a variety of skill levels and training intensities to help children progress (Heyward 2010). Generally, though, children will progress naturally as they age because of their physical and psychological development.

Training periodisation

Training periodisation is a term used to explain a training cycle over a period of time—generally the sport's season. In this training period there may be a preparatory phase, a competition phase and a transition phase. Training periodisation becomes more pertinent when children are older and bracket into competition and is discussed more fully in Chapter 7 (see pp. 100–2).

Individual variability

Children, like adults, have different levels of motivation, fitness and motor skills. You will need to design your training to cater for a range of varying abilities. These can include:

▶ grouping together children with similar abilities and physical development for particular activities or having varying difficulty options

▶ offering closed and open motor skill options

▶ adapting motivational techniques to children's personalities

▶ personalised goal setting.

Diminishing returns

Generally, the more practice a child completes, the greater their performance improvements will be; however, they will reach a point where their performance will plateau and additional training will only create small improvements. Having a child stand on the spot while bouncing a basketball could be a new skill but once they are competent at this they will no longer improve. You will then need to move the child on to the progressive skill of bouncing a basketball while moving. Keeping track of when children have reached competency in a skill and are thus ready to move on to the next skill is part of ensuring that your training sessions are effective.

Reversibility

When a child ceases training they can lose motor skill development and physical adaptations, such as their fitness. A child may go on holidays for one week and this may not affect their fitness or skill level detrimentally. However, if the child has a month off training, a reduction in fitness and skill level can occur. Fitness is generally more likely to be affected than skill level if the skill level prior to the break was high.

The reversibility concept can also be called detraining. Noakes (2003) explained that in adults, fitness can start to fall rapidly in two to three weeks' detraining. Fitness in activities of short duration (5 minutes) is not as negatively affected as longer activities. If one-third of the training program is sustained during the holiday period, most of the aerobic fitness can be retained. Little research has been conducted about children and reversibility effects.

Age

Children have varying levels of physical and psychological development, so training sessions may need to cater for this. It is recommended that:

- for children under the age of 6, exercise is designed to be fun and play-centred with encouragement for being active
- for children aged 6 to 10, guidance is given to develop basic motor skills within a fun environment
- for children aged 11 to 15, more detailed skill techniques and strategies for coping with competition are developed.

It is important to note that children do not have the ability to dissipate and retain heat in the same way that adults do. This means that they are at a far higher risk of heat-related illness. Suggestions on how you can manage this are presented earlier on page 23.

COMPONENTS OF PHYSICAL FITNESS

There are three main components to physical fitness that you need to consider when designing training programs for children (Egger & Champion 1998). These include:

- fitness (aerobic and anaerobic)
- flexibility
- muscle strength.

Ideally, training will incorporate aspects of each of these three areas. However, for different sports there may be a greater focus on one of these components.

Fitness (aerobic and anaerobic)

Improving a child's fitness level is important for most sports. Aerobic fitness (sometimes called cardiovascular fitness) predominately uses the large muscles of the body in movement for an extended period of time, such as when jogging or swimming. In these types of activities the heart and lungs work moderately to supply sufficient oxygen to the body. Children usually feel comfortable during this type of exercise but are not as suited as adults to long, continuous exercise and will need to stop after a period of time.

Aerobic fitness activities are useful in developing efficient hearts, lungs and circulatory systems and aid in improving overall health and weight management. Guiding children to learn techniques for maintaining and improving fitness levels in an enjoyable environment can create positive lifelong habits.

Building anaerobic fitness is particularly useful in short–duration power sports, and sports which have intermittent exercise such as football, netball, tennis and soccer. Training methods for improving anaerobic fitness levels are discussed on the following page.

It is recommended that an aerobic and anaerobic fitness program consist of:

▶ a warm–up
▶ a main section of the session, which usually involves fitness and skill-based activities
▶ a cool-down.

Before stretching, a warm–up consisting of light exercise is recommended. This could be a light jog or similar activity. It is a good idea for the warm–up to focus on the muscles that will be used during the main session. Once this is completed you can introduce stretching. Warming up prior to stretching minimises the risk of injury as the muscles stretch further when warmer.

Once the warm–up is completed, the fitness session can commence. For children, this is usually game- or motor skill-focused at a medium to high intensity, with intermittent short-duration activities. For children up to 12 years of age training sessions usually last around 30 to 45 minutes.

As children become older, their ability for longer endurance events improves, and training sessions of up to an hour or more become safer.

Once the main fitness session is completed the cool-down phase should commence. This consists of slowing the heart rate and completing final stretches. An adequate cool-down will contribute to reducing muscle soreness, increasing flexibility and minimising injury damage and risk.

For adults, a way to check if the intensity of the exercise session is suitable is by performing a rate of perceived exertion (RPE) test. The coach asks how hard the person thinks they are working on a scale of 1 to 10, with 10 being the most intense. Another method for adults is to measure the heart rate by placing two fingers over a pulse—usually at the neck or wrist—and counting the number of beats per minute. These options are not really practical for children as they may not yet be able to take their pulse or accurately read their perceived rate of exertion during exercise. Observation is one of the most effective ways for you to evaluate intensity levels in children. Children are also more likely to stop and train within their limits than adults are.

Types of fitness training

You can use a number of different training methods to add variety to the main section of the fitness training program. These include:

Continuous training

This is the most basic and involves continuous exercise such as swimming or jogging nonstop. As previously mentioned, young children are not as suited to this type of exercise as adults are, so you may need to keep continuous activities relatively short and interspersed rest periods. A maximum of around 10 minutes of continuous exercise is suggested for younger children before they are offered a rest.

Interval training

This type of training is where children exercise for a period of time, such as 30 seconds or 2 minutes, and then rest for a similar period of time. The process is then repeated numerous times over the training session. Interval training is excellent for increasing speed and aerobic and anaerobic fitness levels, and while it can be mentally and physically challenging, the balance between exercise and rest can make it seem more manageable. Interval training should be used with caution as overtraining can occur if the intensity is high and performed too regularly.

Fartlek training

This type of training is similar to interval training though the rest period is replaced with continuing activity of a lower intensity. If a child was running around the oval, they would run fast for 1 minute and then keep jogging at a slower pace during the rest period, with this cycle being repeated a number of times. This training very specifically boosts the anaerobic threshold, which helps improve a child's ability to perform at higher speeds before reaching the point where the body starts going into oxygen debt. Like interval training, fartlek training needs to be used with caution and balance to avoid overtraining and injuries. This type of training is very intense and demanding and should be limited in its use with children.

Circuit training

Circuit training involves setting up exercise stations and having children move around the stations in a continuous manner. There could be a skipping rope at one station and a basketball to bounce at another. This training is fun, adds variety and can be useful in incorporating a large number of different exercises during one training session. It may not be suitable for very young children as they may find it difficult to remember what each station's activities are, even if this is explained and the activity written at each station.

Assessment of aerobic fitness

There are many ways to test an adult's aerobic fitness level but for children a more simplistic approach can be taken. You can ask children to perform continuous exercise for around 4 to 6 minutes and then calculate the distance to measure improvements. Completing this aerobic fitness assessment at the start of the season, about midway through the season and then about four weeks prior to the main competition can offer information used to adapt aerobic fitness training. The measurement from the start of the season to mid-season should show a marked improvement in aerobic fitness. The measurement four weeks prior to the main competition should show if fitness needs to be maintained or some higher intensity work should be incorporated to increase fitness to reach a peak level for competition. It can be difficult to accurately assess children's fitness levels as improvements could be from training or because the child's heart, lungs and other physical systems are developing. Some coaches choose not to conduct fitness assessments and instead work on observational fitness techniques as their assessment method. This is unobtrusive and suitable for children.

Flexibility

The aim of incorporating stretching exercises that increase flexibility is to help children expand and maintain their range of movement to minimise the risk of injury. Children usually have better flexibility than adults. Body temperature can have an impact on flexibility. The warmer the body temperature, the more flexible a child can be, which is why a warm-up is important before stretching. Another factor affecting flexibility is the sex of the child. Normally girls are more flexible than boys, even at a young age.

Types of flexibility exercises

There are four types of flexibility exercises: static stretches, dynamic stretches, ballistic stretches and proprioceptive neuromuscular facilitation (PNF) stretches (Nieman 2007).

Static stretches

Static stretches are those held in one position for around 30 seconds. This type of stretching is commonly used in the cool-down phase.

Dynamic stretches

Dynamic stretches are performed in a slow, steady motion throughout the exercise, for example swinging a leg straight out in front to symbolise a football kick then swinging it back. These types of stretches are incorporated in most warm-up programs.

Ballistic stretches

Ballistic stretching is when the child bounces at the peak of the stretch. This type of stretching is not normally recommended because of the risk of injury. The only time this stretching should be applied is if the child has completed a full warm-up and this activity is required in their sport. If this type of stretching is going to be used, seek professional advice about how to safely teach this stretch.

PNF stretches

This type of stretching is often conducted with the help of another person and involves the other person acting as resistance during the stretch. For example, if a child is lying on the ground and raising one leg for a hamstring stretch, they push the leg in the air towards the ground while the other person pushes the leg up and acts as a resistance. This can create a contract–relax muscle response, which helps improve flexibility and allows the child to take the stretch further. These types of stretches are very common in sports needing a high degree of flexibility, such as gymnastics.

There are numerous books on the market that offer stretching exercises for children, including *Stretching* by Bob Anderson (2000). When teaching children how to stretch, it is important to explain that it is not a competition and they should stretch slowly and to a point where they can feel the muscle stretching but not strong pain (Anderson 2000).

Muscular strength

Muscular strength training is not limited to weight training. There are also a number of other effective strength and conditioning techniques to improve muscular strength in children.

Strength training for children can involve:

- ▶ core-strengthening exercises such as abdominal sit-ups and many Pilates-type exercises
- ▶ plyometric training, which involves contracting then relaxing the muscle, such as when jumping back and forth over a log, skipping, hopping or doing star jumps. Faigenbaum and Chu (2007) explain that plyometric training can be a safe, fun and effective way of enhancing speed of movement and improving power production. As with all strength and conditioning activities, ensure the intensity and volume are within the child's abilities to minimise the risk of injury.
- ▶ weight training, from the age of 8 if the child uses very light weights (between 1 and 3 kilograms) well within their ability, to perform 8 to 15 repetitions with no more than 6 to 8 exercises. The coach will need to fully understand and teach the correct method of exercise movement (Beihoff & Pop 2009).

Muscle bulk does not occur in prepubescent children. The additional muscle strength comes from improved neural pathway messages.

It is recommended when including strength and conditioning training that:

- ▶ a warm-up and 10 minutes of general fitness training be conducted before the strength and conditioning section so the body is fully warm to assist in avoiding injuries
- ▶ the muscle groups being strengthened have the opposing muscle group also strengthened. This will ensure muscle imbalance does not occur. For example, if the child performs core-abdominal exercises it will be important to also strengthen their lower back muscles. If you do not have background knowledge in strength and conditioning training, seek professional advice.

IMPROVING EXERCISE ADHERENCE

Coaches play a substantial role in helping children develop a positive attitude towards exercise. You can achieve this through offering encouragement and support and by developing fun training activities that are at the correct developmental level.

There are a number of theoretical exercise adherence models that may have practical applications which coaches can use to guide children in enjoying and developing a positive attitude towards exercise, which may in turn help them continue participating in sport. (Heyward 2010; Howley & Franks 2007)

Theories of exercise adherence
Behaviour modification model
This model relates to helping children modify or tailor their behaviour through the use of goal-setting and rewards. For example, children are usually thrilled when they meet the standards of their swimming level and are then upgraded to the next. They know and have reached the goal requirements of the swimming level (goal-setting) and usually receive a certificate (reward) for their efforts. The theory is that children are then motivated to want to achieve the next level.

Having a positive role model also falls within the behaviour modification model. If children look up to you as the coach, they will want to please you and continue developing within the sport, particularly if positive feedback is provided.

Health belief model
This model is based on the premise that people are motivated to exercise because of the desire to have a healthy body and to prevent illness. This method is not as useful for helping to motivate younger children as they do not normally fully understand the health benefits of exercise until they are a bit older, and either wish to avoid excess body weight or experience body image issues.

Social cognitive model
This model relates to the theory that a child is more likely to be enthusiastic and eager to exercise and maintain adherence if they believe

they can achieve the exercise activities set. Thus, it is important to design activities at the child's appropriate level. Positive reinforcement and the use of sporting role models (for children around 11 years of age and older) are both excellent motivators and can contribute to exercise adherence.

Transtheoretical model

This model relates to the readiness of the child to participate in an activity. If the child is contemplating or interested in participating in a sport then they are in the early stages of the transtheoretical model. The child may need encouragement and reassurance to join the sport. If the child has just started the sport, they will need positive reinforcement and enjoyment of the activity before the sport becomes a part of their natural weekly routine, lifestyle and habits. The model suggests this can take six months. After this time, the child is more likely to be willing to commit to and become engaged in regular exercise.

Using technology to promote exercise

Compression garments are useful in helping recovery for adults, especially from intense and endurance exercise. No significant research to date has been conducted on the benefits for children in using compression garments, however, it is possible these could aid recovery in older children starting to exercise more competitively.

SUMMARY

▶ When designing a training session, consider the elements of frequency, duration, intensity and mode of exercise.
▶ When designing a training session, consider the basic principles of specificity, progressive overload, age and individual variability.
▶ Physical components of a training program include fitness (aerobic and anaerobic), flexibility and muscular strength.
▶ Strength and conditioning activities for children can include weight training if conducted under certain conditions.

▶ Plyometric activities are an effective strength and conditioning technique you can use when training children, however, these need to be introduced gradually to minimise the risk of injury.

▶ Include a warm-up of light exercise before stretching so the muscles are warm.

▶ Stretching before the main component of training and competition is important to ensure children are prepared and at minimal risk of sustaining an injury.

▶ Stretching after the main component of training and competition is essential to minimise injury risk, increase flexibility and reduce potential muscle soreness.

▶ Continuous, interval, fartlek and circuit training are all types of fitness training that can be incorporated into a training session for variety and to improve fitness.

▶ Developing training activities that are fun and at the correct developmental level can encourage children's exercise adherence, as can providing encouragement and support.

REFLECTIVE QUESTIONS FOR THE COACH

🐚 Do you know whether the children you coach are participating in other sports? Do you think this makes a difference to them, for example their tiredness or energy levels? Maybe the children you coach have few opportunities to exercise so they are very excited and energetic.

🐚 Do you think the duration of your training sessions is suitable?

🐚 What is the intensity of your training sessions? Does it vary weekly? Does it vary throughout each session?

🐚 Is there progressive overload in the training session?

🐚 Is the sport you coach more aerobic or anaerobic in nature?

🐚 How do you currently improve children's fitness levels? What flexibility activities do you include?

🐚 How do you incorporate stretching in your training sessions? What type of stretching do you teach during the warm-up and cool-down phases? How much light exercise do you think children need to do before starting the stretching phase?

- Do you think the children you coach need strength training activities? If so, what type will you include? What is your view on weight training?
- Have you thought about methods of keeping children involved over the longer term in the sport you coach? Did you find any of the theories of exercise adherence useful?
- What are your thoughts on compression garments for children?

CHAPTER FOUR

COACH COMMUNICATION AND ATHLETE DEVELOPMENT STRATEGIES

This chapter covers two main topics. The first is effective coaching communication strategies and the second is about guiding child athlete development through the sporting system over a period of time.

The first topic—coaching effectiveness—is how you communicate instructions to children and present feedback. You may have great training plans, but if the children you coach are standing around confused or don't know how to correct their mistakes, this can impact their learning and development.

The second topic reflects on whether children should specialise in a sport and how early this should occur. An explanation is presented on this topic together with discussion of Balyi's Long-Term Athlete Development model.

In summary, this chapter outlines:

- effective communication techniques for coaching children
- Balyi's Long-Term Athlete Development model for optimising training in the long term
- research on sport specialisation for children
- safety considerations for children in sport
- parental involvement.

EFFECTIVE COACHING COMMUNICATION SKILLS

Children's cognitive abilities differ from those of adults, so the way that you communicate with children may need to alter slightly. It is important to use clear and simple language. You also need to be aware that children might hear a message but not be able to understand it if it is too complicated. Children have limited sporting and life experience so something you consider self-explanatory may need to be fully explained to a child before they understand.

VAK learning styles

Children, like adults, have learning style preferences. Neil Fleming originally developed the VAK (visual, aural, kinaesthetic) learning style model in 1987 and it is still prominent today (Fleming & Baume 2006). While children may have a preference for one style, they can use more than one as learning tools. As a coach, it is useful to be aware of the different learning styles and incorporate as many of these as possible during training sessions. Interestingly, you may find you favour teaching with one learning style over the others because this is your own learning preference. It is important to ensure that you demonstrate actions, give clear instructions and allow children plenty of time to participate in activities (Pangrazi 2007; Stafford 2011).

Visual learning style

A child a with a visual learning style has a preference for learning through seeing actions, demonstrations, pictures, written instructions and visual aids such as DVDs. For a coach, demonstrating skills is very important to children with this learning preference. An occasional training session showing a video of the sport or a picture of a player in action can also help children with a visual learning style grasp the concepts more effectively.

Aural learning style

A child with an aural learning style has a preference for hearing instructions. What you are saying will be very important to a child with this learning preference.

Kinaesthetic learning style

A child with kinaesthetic learning style has a preference for learning through actually performing the exercise. These children prefer minimal instruction and like to get started as soon as possible and learn by doing. They make lots of mistakes through this learning process, but they usually adapt quickly, especially if guided with supportive corrective feedback.

Active listening

Being able to instruct and explain to children what you want them to do is important and an essential communication skill. The other side to communication is being approachable and able to listen to children when they speak to you. This may take patience, as some children may not be able to clearly express what they want. You may need to clarify that you understand correctly (Pangrazi 2007).

Non-verbal communication

Non-verbal communication is made up of the messages you present that are not spoken. Children are sensitive to your non-verbal communication; your body language can tell them whether you are happy or upset with their performance. You may say to a child that making a mistake does not matter, however, if you do so with crossed arms, an angry face or a raised tone of voice, then they will read these signals and know that your words are not expressing how you really feel. Another example is telling a child to forget about an umpire's decision, but throwing your arms in the air and talking angrily. Your body language demonstrates the real message, regardless of the words.

Strong body language can also be used in positive ways. Children being disruptive can sometimes be guided back on track by a simple look in their direction and stern body language.

Presenting effective instructions

Gearity (2012) interviewed athletes to find out what they thought were the three most prominent characteristics of the worst coaches they had experienced. The most common were:

▶ not providing instruction that helped athletes learn
▶ not tailoring instruction and motivational techniques to individuals
▶ being unknowledgeable about the sport the coach was teaching.

Children benefit from coaches focusing on different instructional advice at different stages of their motor skill development. For example, in the cognitive (first) stage of motor skill development, children will need substantial corrective feedback—which is a specific explanation on how to correct technique, together with positive encouragement (Pangrazi 2007). As children's motor skills develop, they still need corrective feedback but not to the same extent. More details on instructional techniques related to the stages of motor skill development are presented in Chapter 1 (see p. 5).

A motor skill's organisation and complexity can influence the type of instructions required too. Skills with high organisation, such as a jump shot in basketball, need the instructions and practice of the activity to be taught as a whole. More details about motor skill organisation and complexity are also presented in Chapter 1 (see p. 1).

The ages of the children being coached influence the level of instructional detail. Very young children have shorter attention spans and need simple, clear and short instructions.

Tailoring instruction and motivational techniques to individuals

Children, like adults, have different personalities, learning styles and backgrounds, so communicating with each child may require a variety of approaches. Some children need extra positive reinforcement when facing a sporting challenge, whereas others are motivated by and enjoy the challenges presented to them. Over time, you will learn each child's personality, but in the early stages there may be some trial and error. The most important thing to remember is that one teaching or motivational style will not always suit every child.

Being knowledgeable about the sport you coach

Most coaches are training children in a sport they have participated in and thus have a good knowledge base. If the sport has facets you are unsure about, there are usually opportunities for you to seek training. Maybe there is an assistant coach or a carer who has specialised knowledge in the area you are concerned about. It can take many years to become a fully proficient coach so do not feel put off asking for assistance.

Feedback

The same study by Gearity (2012) found that athletes described poor coaching techniques as those that offered feedback with little or no value or presented feedback only in negative instances.

After a bad performance, a child's desire to absorb information is lower. Feedback, both positive and constructive, should be regularly given throughout training and competition, not just when a child performs badly. This way, the child is likely to listen to feedback at different situations and times. Remember, children need positive encouragement with a focus on effort and developmental achievements.

Coaching teams

Instructing a group of children to become a coherent team can be a challenge for coaches of team sports. The team with the most talented children does not always win if they cannot work together. Some recommendations to promote team cohesion include:

- ▶ finding common reasons why the children are participating in the sport. Younger children may enjoy the social and friendship element, so encourage and promote these aspects
- ▶ developing team and individual goals
- ▶ explaining what everyone's role is on the team such as being an attacker, a defender or a team captain (Clements n.d.).

BALYI'S LONG-TERM ATHLETE DEVELOPMENT MODEL

Sports scientists use Balyi's Long-Term Athlete Development model (Balyi & Hamilton 2003) as a guide for children's long-term participation in sport. It explains how overall training objectives change and develop with age.

Guidelines for this model have been designed for most sports and are generic. There are some exceptions to the rule, such as the sports in which children start competing at a national and international level at an earlier age, as with gymnastics.

There are four phases to Balyi's Long-Term Athlete Development model.

Phase 1: the fundamental

Estimated age group: boys aged 6 to 9 years and girls aged 5 to 8 years.

The main objectives for coaches setting training for children in this phase are to develop:

▶ fun and play-centred activities
▶ physical capabilities such as fitness, strength, balance and timing
▶ fundamental movement skills for the sport such as jumping, hopping and throwing.

It is also useful for children at this stage to be involved in cooperative games rather than competitive games. If you are coaching tennis, for example, ask the children to hit the ball to each other with the aim of seeing how many hits they can do consecutively. This way the children are working together rather than competing against each other. The competitive element can be introduced later, when children are more emotionally and psychologically developed to handle competition stress.

Phase 2: learning to train

Estimated age group: boys aged 9 to 12 years and girls aged 8 to 11 years.

The main objective for coaches teaching children in this phase is to introduce them to the fundamental skills of the sport. In Phase 1, the focus was on developing the basics of fundamental motor skills such as jumping, hopping and throwing. In Phase 2, the skills are transferred into a sporting context. For example, if you are coaching soccer, the training will start to involve:

▶ learning sport-specific ball skills such as kicking goals
▶ introducing sport-specific fitness activities such as short sprints and sidestepping to simulate running zigzag down the field.

For this age group, the training is more tailored to what children will be doing in sporting competition, however, only a small proportion of training should be competition-focused at this point. Keep training fun and the pressure low.

Phase 3: training to train

Estimated age group: boys aged 12 to 16 years and girls aged 11 to 15 years.

The main objectives for coaches teaching children in this phase are to focus on developing:

▶ physical capabilities, such as aerobic conditioning, to their potential
▶ refined fundamental motor skills central to the sport.

You should also assist children with competition management and motivational tactics to keep children participating in sport. Chapter 5 provides further information on this topic.

In addition, children around this age can start to develop substantial physical differences from their peers. You may need to cater to and amend motivational tactics for children at both ends of the developmental spectrum.

As children develop at different rates, performance outcome may be influenced by developmental growth rather than being based solely on skills. A child who has not yet reached their full height may experience lower performance in a high-jump competition than a child far taller, even if both have similar skill levels. If a child is experiencing slower developmental growth compared to their peers, it is important to continue encouraging them to participate and develop their skills. When the child's growth aligns with their peers they may become more evenly matched, but they will be disadvantaged if they received fewer opportunities for practice and competition because of their slower development. Even if a child does not excel, creating lifelong motor skills and enjoyment of exercise is still a healthy and positive outcome that you can help children achieve.

At the other end of the scale, children who develop earlier than their peers find they usually excel at sport. This can create a very positive experience for these children, who normally go on to enjoy sport throughout their lives. However, in some circumstances, there reaches a time when their peers' development aligns more with theirs, which can result in them no longer excelling. At this stage, it is important to provide additional positive encouragement along with teaching technical and tactical skills that are not as reliant on developmental growth.

Phase 4: training to compete

Estimated age group: boys aged 16 to 18 years and girls aged 15 to 17 years.

The main objectives for coaching children in this phase are to:

- prepare children for competition by designing training programs which help them gain optimal fitness levels
- establish a high standard of sport-specific skills.

Evaluation of competition performance and competitors can also come into play to help you determine how to structure and focus training for individuals and teams. Particular weaknesses of the children you are coaching may become apparent in competition, so reflecting on this can help you tailor your training sessions to improve on these specific needs. Training can also incorporate a focus on strategy and tactical skill development. These should still always be presented in an encouraging and learning-focused environment.

INFLUENCE OF AGE ON THE TRAINING PROGRAM

The age of a child can impact the type and level of training you design for them. Age is usually thought of as a child's chronological age, which is taken from the day they were born. However, a child can also be classified by biological, developmental and training ages, each of which can affect their ability to perform sporting activities.

Biological age

A child's biological age relates to their physical maturity. This means that while two children can have a chronological age of 10, one may have physically developed earlier and be classed with the physical maturity of a 12-year-old. This can cause problems if these two children are matched in contact sports or even in individual sports, as the child who has not physically matured as early may be at a disadvantage. Helping match children more with their biological age or weight category for their age in contact sports or training activities can also help reduce the risk of injuries. Providing encouragement to those children less physically mature to keep active and continue developing motor skills is important, as these children may later develop and be just as good as, if not better than, their peers.

Developmental age

A child's developmental age is a combination of their biological age (physical maturity) and their emotional and social development. You may find that a child looks physically more mature than other children, however, their emotional and social development may not yet be as advanced. Children with lower emotional and social development levels may lack self-confidence and may experience trouble dealing with social groups and the pressures of competition. As a coach, you need to establish techniques to assist children to cope with the pressures associated with competition. A review of Chapter 5 will provide ways to help children deal with stress and anxiety. If a child has a higher developmental age than their chronological age, you may be able to move them forward in their athletic training model without causing undue stress and strain.

Training age

A child's training age is the number of years they have participated in that sport. The principle is that generally the longer a child has been participating in a sport, the more likely they are to cope with more advanced training sessions.

You may have a team of 10-year-olds but within this group you may have children with a range of biological, development and training ages. This can influence the way training is structured, such as how you pair children together in activities and the variety of activity difficulty levels you'll need to offer.

In general, the biological age (physical maturity of a child) has the greatest impact on performance output, followed closely by the training age of a child.

As children grow, their spatial awareness and coordination can be affected and they may become clumsy at certain stages in their growth. This is because children's body sections grow in different proportions—a child's head will grow to about twice its birth size, whereas their legs will grow about five times their birth size.

Accelerated growth is usually greatest during adolescence. This commonly commences in girls aged 10 to 12 and boys aged 12 to 14.

When children reach this developmental stage, their bodies expend extra energy to support growth. As a result, you may need to focus on skill development at training and less on high-intensity and long-duration fitness activities to minimise placing extra stress and energy expenditure on the child during this phase.

Prior to adolescence, girls and boys have minimal skeletal differences, however, during and after adolescence, girls will experience an increase in hip width and boys change in trunk proportion. Some girls will then become more susceptible to lower-body injuries and boys may experience more balance problems. Girls usually also experience an increase in body fat whereas boys may experience a reduction in body fat. This can make girls more susceptible to weight management concerns. Sensitivity and nutritional support may be required from you when dealing with these issues.

SPORT SPECIALISATION

Specialisation involves focusing on one activity over a period of time in order to become efficient and practiced at that activity. Some coaches (and carers) are concerned that if a child does not specialise in one sport early on, they will not have the opportunity to become highly proficient at that sport. What has actually been found is that if children specialise and train too intensely too early (usually prior to 15 years of age) then they will be more likely to drop out of the sport, experience injuries and overtraining symptoms, and possibly be affected emotionally by not being able to cope with the stress of intense training and competition (Baker, Cobley & Thomas 2009; Cross & Lyle 1999).

Having children participate in a range of sports is not detrimental to their potential for reaching the elite level. It is not until the mid-teenage years that children need to specialise and start to train intensely if they choose to do so (Moesch et al. 2011). Balyi's Long-Term Athlete Development model (see p. 59) is a good basis for coaches training children to determine which focus objectives should occur at different ages to promote longevity in sport.

Training for children should be fun, games-based and focused on skill development. If children are given the opportunity to develop their skills in a fun, non-competitive environment they will be more able to cope with the intensity of training later on.

The only exceptions are those sports in which children need to perform nationally and internationally at very young ages, such as gymnastics. Even then, elite performance commences around the early teenage years for girls, who generally develop earlier than boys.

This does not mean that children cannot participate from an early age in the sport they go on to achieve in at the highest level. This is still a good idea; it is more that the training should not be for a sole sport conducted at the intensity of an adult's program.

One of the greatest challenges for coaches is keeping children participating in a sport long enough to develop the necessary skills and fitness. Ensuring the training is not too intense too soon is one of the ways you can influence the attrition (dropout) rate of children from their sport.

ENSURING SAFETY

The safety of the children in your care is imperative. You can help support the safety of children by analysing the playing area and safety equipment and structuring the training program to minimise injuries. Safety also extends to emotional safety. This means each child should have the opportunity to train feeling safe from bullying and taunts from other children.

Some tactics to promote an emotionally positive training environment include:

▶ having children partner up and requesting that one child in the partnership present positive feedback on how their partner performed a sporting activity. A child may say 'well done' to their partner for hitting their tennis serve within the service box. This task means that while one child is occupied performing a task, the other is occupied reviewing a performance. The review process offers a learning experience for both children and is a way to promote positive encouragement

▶ promote sportsmanship and fair play by rewarding these either through external rewards or positive praise such as highlighting when a child offers some encouraging words

▶ setting up a fair-play sports board which rewards children with a sticker or similar for behaviour you want to promote, such as not arguing with a referee.

PARENTAL INVOLVEMENT

Parental influence is strong among children. Hedstrom and Gould (2004) explain that carers can affect a child's motivation, perceived competence, enjoyment and anxiety about sport. A carer's feedback and behaviour can also influence how long a child will stay in the sport. A study of 154 high-school coaches by Gould, Chung et al. (2006) found coaches reported problems with carers as one of the most frequent issues they had to deal with. In a similar study of junior tennis coaches conducted by Gould, Lauer et al. (2006), the coaches believed 36% of the carers hurt their child's tennis development, and 59% of the carers had a positive influence on their child's tennis development.

'Ugly parent syndrome' is the term used when carers become highly vocal and disruptive. The carer is too focused on the results of a match or the child's performance and bellows negative comments to the child, officials, coaches or other carers.

Hedstrom and Gould (2004) summarised the five biggest carer–child interaction problems as:

- overemphasising winning
- holding unrealistic expectations
- coaching one's own child
- criticising one's own child
- pampering the child too much.

Recommendations to combat these problems and the 'ugly parent syndrome' include:

- giving referees and officials the power to send spectators from the field
- establishing ground rules (including a code of conduct) with carers prior to the season commencing
- introducing penalty points for improper spectator behaviour or bonus points for positive spectator behaviour (Department of Sport and Recreation 2003).

It is important where possible for you as a coach to develop a positive relationship with carers. The majority of carers do positively influence their child's sporting development and children love making their carers happy. You should advise carers about the positive achievements their child makes, emphasising the child's developmental progress rather than winning outcomes. Hopefully, this will result in carers giving positive feedback to their children and emphasising their developmental progress rather than winning.

Carers have also been known to influence a child's anxiety levels before, during and after competition. Teaching children anxiety management techniques (covered in Chapter Five) can assist in these situations.

Parental involvement is useful for coaches, because in many circumstances you will need volunteers to keep the sport going. Ensure you are approachable for carers. Communicate with them about their children and, if they are interested in helping, how best they can assist. Some organisations have:

- a code of conduct for carers
- an orientation day at the start of the season
- a newsletter emphasising the coaching philosophy about children having fun, skill development progress and any social events.

One of the greatest challenges for carers is accepting their child's abilities. Not every child will go on to be an elite athlete. There are, however, many other wonderful attributes that can be taken from participation in sport, including motor skill development, social skills development, teamwork development and health benefits. These should be emphasised throughout training and communicated with carers.

Moral responsibilities

Children will look up to you as a coach for guidance not just in their sporting development but also in how you conduct yourself. Children learn and sometimes mimic adult behaviour so it is important to ensure you are a positive role model for the children you coach.

SUMMARY

- Children's cognitive abilities differ from adults', so the way you communicate will need to alter slightly.
- When communicating with children, you need to use clear and simple language.
- Children have limited sporting and life experience and thus limited frames of reference, so do not assume they will automatically understand tasks that you see as self-evident.
- Children have different learning style preferences, such as aural, visual and kinaesthetic, so offering different communication techniques can help bridge the gap of communication.
- Effective instructional techniques involve giving specific feedback, tailoring instruction and motivational techniques to individuals and being knowledgeable about the sport and how children can improve.

▶ Balyi's Long-Term Athlete Development model has four phases of development and is recommended as a coaching tool to improve the longevity of children's participation in sport. Each phase has training objectives on which you can base children's training goals.

▶ The age of children can influence training programs. You should consider not only a child's chronological age but their biological, developmental and training ages as well.

▶ You are responsible for the safety of the children you teach. This means ensuring that the equipment and playing fields are safe, the training techniques and activities are safe and the training is conducted in an emotionally safe learning environment.

▶ Carers have a significant influence on children's motivation, perceived competence, enjoyment and anxiety about sport.

▶ Communicate with carers about how important they are to their children's sporting development and how best they can help you and their child achieve enjoyment and development in sport.

REFLECTIVE QUESTIONS FOR THE COACH

✎ Using the VAK learning style model, what do you think is your own preferred learning style? Of the three, how many learning style techniques would you be incorporating in training sessions throughout the season? Could you incorporate any of the given VAK learning style examples at your training?

✎ How often do you give feedback? Do you tend to use feedback more for encouragement or more for corrective purposes? Do you think your feedback is influenced by the age of the children you coach?

✎ How often is your feedback distributed to the group as a whole or to individual children? Do you need to tailor your instructions and motivational techniques for individual children?

✎ At what phase of Balyi's Long-term Athlete Development model are the children you coach? How close are your coaching objectives to the model's recommendations? What is the average national competition age for children or adults in the sport you coach?

- At what age do you think children should specialise in your sport? When does the training start to become intense?
- What is the attrition rate of children dropping out of the sport? What do you think the reasons are for this?
- Are the children you coach very different in biological, developmental and training ages? Do you use any techniques to cater for these differences?
- What are the carers of the children you coach like? How do you involve the carers?
- How do you report progress or information about the children to the carers?
- Do any of the carers have useful skills that could assist you?
- How do you deal with difficult carers?

CHAPTER FIVE

SPORTS PSYCHOLOGY FOR COACHING CHILDREN

This chapter explains how you can use sport psychology to assist children in developing a positive attitude towards exercise and help them cope with the competitiveness involved in sport.

Children's participation in sport can affect their self-concept (perception of self) and self-esteem (perception of their value as a person). Younger children are not normally aware of their competencies, however, as they grow older, they start comparing themselves with others and evaluating what people central to their lives think of their performance. As a coach, you need to be aware that the way you structure your training, how you motivate children, how you react to their performance and the feedback you give can have a substantial impact on how children view themselves in relation to sport and exercise.

This chapter covers:

▶ motivational techniques to increase children's enjoyment in sport participation
▶ motivational theories and their practical implications for coaches
▶ techniques to help children manage anxiety
▶ visualisation and goal-setting techniques to enhance confidence and motivation
▶ gender and motivation.

MOTIVATIONAL TECHNIQUES

Motivation is what drives a person and compels them to action. Children are usually keen to participate in exercise so motivating them to join in the activities is not normally a problem. However, it is important that you create positive exercise experiences as these can influence whether the children continue with the sport and can affect their exercise participation later on in life.

Fun and game-centred activities

It is important that training for younger children is centred on fun and game-like activities. You can develop a child's motor skills and fitness while encouraging the fun, social and team elements within group games such as tunnel ball and relay running (Australian Sports Commission 2008).

Exercise should not be used as a punishment

It is highly recommended that exercise not be used as punishment. If a child is misbehaving, do not make them run laps or do ten push-ups. Participating in exercise should be a rewarding experience. Lavay et al. (2011) found that the most common methods for managing disruptive behaviour during physical education classes for children are the use of: time-out, direct discussion, planned ignoring of the behaviour and verbal reprimands.

Select the teams

As a coach, select the teams yourself. Avoid two team captains selecting children and leaving the last few noticeably waiting to be chosen. This is not conductive to enhancing self-esteem and focuses on 'best friends' and talent.

Create exercise achievement

If children are able to achieve tasks, this will boost their self-esteem and encourage them to continue. One of your challenges is to set activities at the correct level for the children and to offer a range of task difficulties to suit the varying levels within the group. Children should feel a sense of satisfaction about their participation at the end of each training session.

Understand why children exercise

Halls (n.d.), the senior regional coordinator of the Active After School Communities Program, stated in a *Sports Coach* article that children exercise to:

- have fun
- develop fitness
- make friends
- learn new skills
- enjoy competition
- be challenged.

If you understand their reasons, you can incorporate as many elements as possible to motivate children to exercise and continue participating in the sport.

MOTIVATIONAL THEORIES AND THEIR PRACTICAL APPLICATION

Motivational theories have been developed to guide understanding about why and how people are motivated. A brief outline of these theories and how you can apply them in a practical setting when coaching children follows.

Extrinsic and intrinsic motivation

Extrinsic and intrinsic motivation relate to the source of motivation. Extrinsic motivation includes rewards presented from external sources, such as when a child exercises because they want to please their carers and coaches or to win the first-place blue ribbon. This type of motivation can be strong within children. Certificates of participation can be useful as encouragement tools, particularly when children are just beginning and not experiencing high performance outcomes. Extrinsic motivation can also simply be skill-development-focused praise from you, such as, 'That's a fantastic ball toss—it was high and just slightly forward of the body. Well done!'

Intrinsic motivation drives children to exercise for their own personal reasons. The social side of sport can be a strong intrinsic motivational factor—one of the most common examples is a child asking their carer if they can play the same sport as their friends. Other intrinsic motivations include children enjoying the exercise, having a positive learning environment or participating in the end-of-year sports performance day. You can help develop children's intrinsic motivation by arranging positive and fun exercise experiences, providing activities children feel competent at, encouraging team group events and socialising during the breaks, and discovering and encouraging children's strengths. Intrinsic motivation is important to develop because as children grow older, the likelihood of them being showered with external motivators such as ribbons, certificates and stickers for participation usually reduces. As children become adults, their desire to please their carers and coaches diminishes, too, so again, it is important to develop their intrinsic motivation to exercise.

Achievement motivation

Achievement motivation is the sense of satisfaction received from reaching a goal. Children are motivated by numerous reasons to commence a sport, such as wanting to join because their friend or their big brother is doing the sport. However, children will remain motivated in the sport if they feel a sense of achievement from either their own point of view or the view of someone they admire, such as a coach or carer. Praise can be a very powerful tool in helping motivate a child to train. In some circumstances, especially in the early stages of motor skill learning, the child will not achieve great success. You will need to set tasks that children can reach and feel like they have made some progress and achieved (Anshel 2011).

To assist a child's motivation through achievement, it is recommended that you:

▶ allocate tasks that children find challenging yet are able to achieve or get close to achieving. You may need to set different difficulty levels to cater for varied abilities
▶ provide corrective yet encouraging feedback on how children can improve their skills
▶ remind children of progress made and that their skill levels are improving and will continue to do so
▶ provide continual encouragement.

It is also important that if a child is not good at a sport, they do not start to develop the thought that this is true of all sports. Sports have varying requirements of fitness levels, balance, flexibility, reaction time, strength and many other factors, and different children will naturally be better at different sports.

Competency motivation theory

This theory is similar to achievement theory in that children and adults usually continue with something they feel competent at. Including a mixture of activities that are individual and group-based will allow children who are not as strong to be part of a team that does well. Even for individual sports such as swimming, arranging relay activities with a mixture of swimming levels is a good way to even out the competition (Anshel 2011).

Within this theory is also the concept of perceived competence. A child may be adequate at certain skills, however, the people around them—perhaps a carer—may not be giving them positive feedback about their skill development. A child may not have to ability to understand and assess their own skill level and sometimes the high expectations of others can make them feel they are not competent, when in fact they are. You can help children learn about their own competency levels if you point out when they are performing a skill or aspects of a skill correctly.

MANAGING ANXIETY BEFORE AND DURING EXERCISE

A fear of failure and creating disappointment in the people a child loves and respects can have a profound effect on a child's performance and enjoyment of exercise.

Anxiety is created when a child perceives a negative difference between the skills they have and the demands of a situation. It results in a fight-or-flight response involving an elevated heart rate, muscle tension and a release of adrenaline, which in turn can drain energy after the adrenaline has been released. Anxiety can prepare the body for action, which can be useful in a sporting event. The key to anxiety is getting the level correct; that is, creating enough anxiety and challenge to boost the body to prepare for exercise.

Sports psychologists call this balance of adrenaline and anxiety the 'arousal performance curve', drawn as a bell shape. The ideal anxiety level is at the peak of the curve, so a child benefits from the positive effects of the fight-or-flight response, without becoming too anxious and reducing their performance ability (McMorris 2004). If a child believes the goal is unachievable, then the anxiety may overextend, possibly resulting in the child losing interest in participating, not trying, getting upset, being rebellious or feeling tired throughout the performance. If a child begins to show symptoms of being unable to concentrate or if their skill levels (especially fine motor movements) are affected, they will need to undertake techniques to reduce their anxiety.

All children respond differently to anxiety before a sporting event. You could have two children with very similar skill abilities who may perceive the participation in the sport differently. One child may enjoy a pep talk to get them all fired up, whereas the other child may need anxiety management techniques to calm them down. You will need to assess each child's anxiety levels and what techniques best suit them.

The type of exercise and sport the child is participating in can affect the desired level of anxiety. Shorter, more explosive events can allow for a greater level of anxiety to be experienced—the extra adrenaline will help in a 100-metre sprint, for example. Events using fine motor skills, such as archery, require a lower level of anxiety, to keep hands steady.

Sport and competition have been found to be useful for teaching children how to deal with adversity, make new friends, work in a team environment and build self-esteem. Competition can also teach them that they cannot be the best at everything and how to deal with this.

Factors influencing anxiety

Factors affecting the level of anxiety a child will experience before participating in a sporting activity can include:

▶ the importance of the event. Bigger events, such as school carnivals or interstate competitions, will likely cause a child to become more anxious
▶ the readiness of a child to physically and psychologically participate in the sport. Children develop motor skill abilities and mental conditioning at different ages, and placing them in a situation beyond their capabilities will be stressful for them
▶ the personality of the child. Some personality types are more prone to higher expectations of themselves and a stronger desire to win
▶ external support for the child. Children who have supportive carers and coaches encouraging them will feel less anxious.

Alleviating anxiety

There are a number of techniques, described below, that you can use to help children alleviate anxiety.

Progressive muscular relaxation

This technique involves relaxing one muscle at a time. You might ask the child to start at their feet, clench each foot and then relax it. You then move to the calf muscles. Ask the child to focus on tightening each calf muscle and then relaxing it. When a person becomes anxious, their muscles tighten. This technique works by releasing the tension in the muscles.

Positive imagery

This technique is about visualising a happy and positive place. Ask the child to stop and focus on producing an image in their mind of a place where they feel calm and at peace. These peaceful thoughts help promote calmness, relaxation of the muscles and to return to breathing to a more composed pace.

The four-breath technique

This technique involves having the child focus their attention on their breathing. When a child becomes anxious they take shallower, more rapid breaths. The aim is to regain control of the breathing, making it steadier and from the diaphragm. A child can achieve this by taking one big breath in and then exhaling. The focus should be on counting to four while breathing in and then counting to four while breathing out. So the breath in should take four counts and the breath out four counts. It also helps by having the child place their hand on their stomach just above the level of their belly button and getting them to focus on moving their hand in and out as the diaphragm moves with their breathing. This helps the child draw a deeper breath.

Keeping winning in perspective

Both children and adults like to win. It is important that children understand that while they may dislike losing, it is not a reflection of them as a whole. They still have many positive skills and attributes as a person. In addition, one event will not usually affect a child's total sporting career, so as a coach you can help children see this perspective.

Control the controllable

This technique is about helping to alleviate anxiety by guiding the child to focus on controllable events and not get worked up about those events they cannot control. For example, a list can be made about whether the cause of anxiety is a controllable or an uncontrollable issue. If it is uncontrollable, such as the weather or the decisions of the umpire, then the child needs to let go of any energy or anxiety about this aspect. Instead, teach children to focus their energy and anxiety on things they can control, such as their practice sessions, breathing techniques and their own performance.

Energetic warm-up

An energetic warm-up can help children expel some of their nerves. The exercising will help them breathe more heavily and get their muscles moving, releasing any tension that is building up.

Music

Listening to music can be helpful for some children in alleviating anxiety. It can switch their mind off the activity and can be a powerful motivational tool. Music can also be tailored to whether the child needs to calm down or is interested in becoming more energised.

Similarity of preparation

If children have a similar warm-up for training and competition, the familiarity of this task prior to the event can help soothe their anxiety. Some children also wear the same outfit or have the same meal to establish this familiarity and create calmness.

VISUALISATION AND GOAL-SETTING TECHNIQUES

Visualisation

Visualisation is a technique where children imagine themselves performing a skill or routine in a successful way. Visualisation is thought to work effectively through two different means. The first is that when a child performs a practical activity, their memory stores the sensory experience. When the child visualises the activity, it allows them to regain a sense of the memory and practise creating positive repetition in their mind, which contributes to building self-confidence. The second idea is that during visualisation, the mind can recall the motor pathways of the physical activity being rehearsed through either the central nervous system being activated or through a symbolic method of learning (Shaw, Gorely & Corban 2005). Either way, visualisation can effectively help children:

▶ remember their skill or routine performed in a successful way
▶ build self-confidence through the repetition of successful performance
▶ enhance motor pathways to remember successful performance.

If you choose to teach visualisation techniques, suggest that the child:

▶ use as many senses as possible during the visualisation—visualise in colour, how they felt during practice and what it sounded like
▶ go through the components of the activity step-by-step
▶ visualise performing the activity successfully.

While visualisation has been found to be beneficial, this technique alone will not create dramatic improvements. Visualisation is an accompanying technique to help children improve performance, particularly:

▶ in activities involving routines with many skill aspects, such as complex gymnastic routines
▶ for improving confidence
▶ by reducing performance anxiety.

It is also more suitable for older children.

Goal-setting

Goal-setting is a technique used to initiate and maintain changes in behaviour. Helping children to set goals can motivate them to train regularly and, when they become older, at intensity. Goals help provide a focus and a target which is measureable, giving children a sense of achievement at meeting objectives. The goals set should be challenging yet achievable, and will depend on the child's age, their ability and also what they want to achieve.

Examples of goal-setting for children include:

▶ to beat their 100-metre sprint time within the next four competitions
▶ to make the state soccer team in the next year
▶ to achieve a higher percentage of first serves within the service box during the next tennis season.

Some of these goals may be short-term and others longer-term. It is a good idea to have a mixture of short- and long-term goals, however, younger children are more suited to short-term goals as they have difficulty thinking much beyond the immediate future.

Designing goals

It is recommended that only a few goals be made. Having too many can be confusing for a child and can mean losing the clarity that goal-setting has to offer.

While most goals for children will be performance-based, goal-setting can also help them to focus on the mental side of exercise, such as using techniques to reduce their anxiety before competition from a 9 to a 7 out of 10.

Where possible, it is recommended that most goals focus on a child's self-improvement. This is more under a child's control and can reduce anxiety about the unknown abilities of other competitors. As children become older, more goals involving competition with others can be introduced if you and the child decide this is appropriate.

There are a number of principles to remember when designing exercise goals, which form the acronym SMART: specific, measurable, attainable, realistic and time-specific.

Specific

Outline as much detail as possible in the goal, for example, to beat a personal best time in the 100-metre sprint within the next four competitions.

Measureable

The goal needs to be set so that the child will be able to tell clearly if they have achieved it.

Attainable

The goal should be challenging so the child will have to strive for it and will feel satisfaction at achieving success. If the goal is too far beyond their reach and abilities then negative anxiety will set in, which can be detrimental to the child's motivation. Perhaps the child has already beaten their personal best time for the 100 metres on a number of occasions during the season. To beat it again might be too difficult in such a short time frame.

Goals should also be set with the child in mind. As a coach, you may have your own goals but it is important to remember not to force your goals onto a child. A child may not want to train seven days a week to make the state or international team. Goals need not always be grand in scale.

Realistic

Realistic goals are similar in concept to attainable goals. You need to evaluate a child's ability, age and motivation when helping them set goals. The goals should be achievable not only in your mind but in the child's mind too.

Time

The goal should have a time frame to assist in the drive to complete the goal.

GENDER AND MOTIVATION

Sometimes coaches can be affected by the stereotype of the sport they teach. It is important that regardless of which sport you coach, you:

- avoid gender-stereotypical comments
- have similar expectations of performance for both girls and boys. Particularly in the earlier years, children of both sexes have minimal differences in strength, endurance and physical skills
- recognise that personality can influence exercise preference—some children are more competitive than others
- present encouraging feedback focused on skill development regardless of the sex of the child. Boys need encouragement and positive reinforcement as much as girls do. Coaching boys should not be more outcome-focused than coaching girls (Pangrazi 2007).

SUMMARY

- Children enjoy exercising because it is fun, they develop new skills, they have opportunities to play sport with their friends and they are challenged.
- Extrinsic motivational tactics are the provision of external rewards such as ribbons, certificates and praise.
- Intrinsic motivations are personal reasons why children want to participant in sport, such as being excited about joining their friends, training for the big performance or learning how to bowl in cricket. You can promote children's intrinsic motivation through developing fun training sessions, promoting group game activities and conducting training at a level they find challenging, interesting and achievable.
- Anxiety before competition can be influenced by the importance of an event, a child's personality, their readiness for the event and their external support network.

- To reduce anxiety before competition, eight techniques are outlined, including keeping winning in perspective, similarity in preparation and the four-breath technique.
- Visualisation is an effective accompanying mental tool to improving self-esteem, confidence and performance.
- Goal-setting can be used to improve focus and motivation. The goals should be designed using the SMART principles.

REFLECTIVE QUESTIONS FOR THE COACH

- What are the main reasons you think the children you coach are participating in the sport?
- What extrinsic motivational techniques are used in your sport? Are there certificates, ribbons, trophies? Do the children want to please you and their carers?
- What are the most effective motivational techniques you think your sport has?
- Do you think the difficulty level of training is achievable for the children? What techniques are used to make the level easier or harder? How competitive are the children you coach?
- How anxious are the children you coach before competition? Which of the eight anxiety-reducing techniques would you prefer to incorporate in your coaching?
- Do you think using visualisation and goal-setting would be beneficial for your group of children? If so, how would you incorporate it?

SPORTS NUTRITION FOR CHILDREN

You can teach children and advise carers about the most effective foods and fluid to consume before, during and after exercise to maintain children's energy levels and improve their recovery.

This chapter outlines:

▶ the food nutrients, describing what they are and how they help the body during exercise
▶ recommended food and fluid consumption before and during exercise
▶ food and fluids that promote recovery after exercise
▶ the latest research on sports drinks for children.

FOOD NUTRIENTS

Carbohydrates

Carbohydrates are a critical source of fuel for a child's body. The more exercise children undertake, the greater their need to replenish their carbohydrate stores. When carbohydrates are consumed, they are broken down in the body and stored as blood glycogen. Small amounts of blood glycogen are stored within a child's liver and a larger amount is stored within the muscles. When children exercise, blood glycogen from the liver and muscle stores is broken down to create blood glucose, which is used to create energy. There is enough blood glycogen stored in an adult's muscles to last for between 60 and 90 minutes of exercise. Little research has been conducted on children's blood glycogen stores and usage during exercise, so we have to work on a similar assumption of blood glucose depletion as for adults.

Most training sessions for children last less than 60 to 90 minutes, so carbohydrate loading (consuming high levels of carbohydrates before exercise) is not essential for children. However, children will need to replace the carbohydrate stores lost during exercise. The best way to do this is explained later in this chapter (see p. 93).

When a child wakes in the morning, the blood glycogen stores in their liver have diminished. It is therefore important, especially if the child will be exercising in the morning, that they consume food and fluids to replenish these blood glycogen stores. Some children find it difficult to eat early in the morning, so some alternative food and fluid suggestions are presented later in this chapter (see p. 91). Replenishing liver glycogen stores is important to avoid 'brain drain'. Glover and Glover (1999) used this term to describe what happens if blood glycogen stores in the liver are low when a child exercises. Rather than transporting full sources to the brain as well as the muscles, the blood glycogen from the muscles is used to create energy, leaving the child feeling groggy and unable to fully concentrate.

In the 1980s, carbohydrates were often divided into the categories of simple and complex. At the time, complex carbohydrates were the recommended source of carbohydrates as these provided a larger amount of dietary fibre, minerals and vitamins. Simple carbohydrates were considered less nutritious as these were higher in sugar content and contained fewer nutrients. During the 1980s, health promotion revolved around choosing wholegrain and wholemeal breads, pastas and rice as opposed to the refined products. Later research described by Burke and Cox (2010) found that the division between complex and simple carbohydrates was not always clear. Some simple carbohydrate foods were found to be more nutritious, so today the division of simple and complex carbohydrates is not as regularly promoted.

In the 1990s, new research found carbohydrate-rich foods had a unique effect on blood glucose. This effect was unrelated to simple and complex carbohydrate groupings and was called the glycaemic index. Carbohydrate foods were categorised according to the rate at which blood glucose was released into the blood stream. Foods releasing blood glucose slowly were deemed to have a low glycaemic index (GI). Foods in this category include apples, pears and low-fat frozen yogurt. Foods that release blood glucose quickly into the body were deemed high-glycaemic foods. Examples of these include sports drinks, cornflakes, lollies and white bread.

It was thought that foods with a low glycaemic index could be eaten before competition to give sustaining energy, whereas foods with a high glycaemic index would be perfect for after training and during competition to restore energy quickly. The majority of recent research, however, as explained by Burke and Cox (2010), has found little difference in performance between pre-event meals of low-GI compared to high-GI foods.

Proteins

Proteins, like carbohydrates, offer the body a source of energy. When proteins are ingested they are broken down into amino acids. These amino acids travel to the liver, where they are stored as blood glycogen and when needed are broken down into blood glucose to create energy. The broken-down protein amino acids also travel to the body's tissues to help create muscle movement during exercise. Protein can be found in meats, fish, eggs, dairy products (milk, cheese and yoghurt), whole grains and cereals, baked beans and nuts. Children have a slightly higher protein need than adults because of their body's growth. Protein helps support bone and tissue development in children.

Protein requirements increase with exercise, due to protein's contribution to creating muscle energy and repairing tissue damage from intense training. Burke and Cox (2010) explain that most children consume enough protein. Protein supplements and powders are definitely not needed or recommended. If you feel children need extra protein, there are many sources of protein available from foods, especially as they can offer additional nutritional benefits. For example, milk contains protein and is also a rich source of calcium.

For children who are vegetarian, it is important to note that plant foods may be missing one or more essential amino acids found in animal-based protein foods. This means they will need a full range of plant and vegetable foods so they gain all the essential amino acids. Vegetarian children should have dairy products such as milk, yoghurt and cheese as well as eggs, nuts, cereals, grains and legumes such as baked beans.

A vegan diet may be suitable for children who are involved in sport, but a consultation with a health professional (e.g. nutritionist) is recommended to ensure they are receiving sufficient quantities of all the vitamins and minerals they need, particularly vitamin B12.

Fats and oils

Fats and oils are in many of our favourite foods. Examples of foods with fats and oils include: milk, cheese, yoghurt, margarine, butter, ice-cream, cakes, meat, nuts and peanut butter. Fats and oils can provide the body with essential fatty acids and fat-soluble vitamins. They can also provide a concentrated source of energy, however, they are not the preferred source of energy for the body during exercise. Food with a high fat content is more likely to have a high sugar content, which can contribute to tooth decay in children. Fats also have twice as many calories per gram than carbohydrates and proteins, so monitoring fat intake for children is important for creating healthy lifetime habits and for some children as weight management. Some foods high in fat and oil can also have minimal dietary fibre, vitamin and mineral content and can be high in saturated fat and trans fatty acids, which are the unhealthier oils. Foods containing high levels of saturated fat and trans fatty acids include deep-fried food, pastries, confectionary and biscuits. In addition, saturated fat and trans fatty acids are present in meat, dairy products, and coconut and palm oils. As meat and dairy products have other health benefits these are promoted as nutritional foods for children. The healthier fat and oil choices are polyunsaturated and mono-unsaturated fats found in olive oil, peanut and canola oils, oily fish, wholegrain cereals and nuts.

Vitamins and minerals

Calcium

Calcium assists with bone formation during a child's growth. Calcium also manages muscle and nerve function. It is recommended children have around 1000 milligrams of calcium per day, which is equivalent to a glass of milk, two slices of cheese, some yoghurt and a few almonds. This is greater than the recommended calcium intake for adults, which is around 800 milligrams (Burke & Deakin 2008). A large-scale survey of Australian children (CSIRO 2008) found that the majority of children in all age groups met the estimated average requirements for all of the assessed nutrients, with the exception of calcium and magnesium. In the case of girls aged 14 to 16 years, between 82 per cent and 89 per cent did not meet the estimated average requirements (CSIRO 2008). This is a cause for concern.

The best sources of calcium include dairy products such as milk, cheese and yoghurt, fish with edible bones, almonds and some green vegetables. If children are lactose intolerant then lactose-reduced milk or calcium-fortified rice or soy beverages are alternatives. Dairy products could cause stomach and digestion problems if consumed before exercise, however, they are excellent food and drink sources to aid recovery after exercise.

Iron

Iron is necessary for children as it produces haemoglobin in their red blood cells. During exercise, haemoglobin carries oxygen from the lungs to the body's muscles and tissues, which aids breathing efficiency. Iron is also essential in creating chemical reactions that produce energy in the body and boosts resistance to disease and stress. A deficiency in iron is called anaemia and can result in symptoms such as fatigue, loss of energy and headaches. Doctors can test children's iron levels and low iron can usually be combated by increasing the number of iron-rich foods within a child's diet.

Iron is found in red meat, poultry, fish and other seafood, legumes such as baked beans, green leafy vegetables, cereals, wholemeal bread and dried fruits. Iron is classified into two types: heme and non-heme. Heme iron is more easily absorbed and has a higher iron count. It is found in some animal foods. Non-heme iron is poorly absorbed and can be affected by the consumption of some foods and drinks, such as tea, wheat bran and wholemeal cereals. Vitamin C can assist in the absorption of non-heme iron, so a glass of orange juice with a child's breakfast cereal can be beneficial.

Girls who have started menstruating have higher iron requirements and will need to ensure they consume enough iron to maintain energy levels (Burke & Deakin 2008).

Water

Water is the most important nutrient for a child. If a child's body is dehydrated, their ability to exercise will be affected. One method of testing for dehydration is for the child to check the colour of their urine. Excluding first thing in the morning, a child's urine should be clear in colour. If this is not the case, the child may not be consuming enough fluids. Vitamin supplements can influence urine colour, so if a child takes vitamins in the morning, they should wait until the afternoon before taking note of the colour of their urine.

Rowland (2011) explains that children may become distracted and forget to consume enough fluids during and after training, so coaches and carers may need to remind them. Rowland's study found that children should consume 13 millilitres of fluids per kilogram of body weight per hour during exercise (about 500 millilitres for a child weighing 40 kilograms), and 4 millilitres of fluids per kilogram per hour of exercise after completing exercise to assist in replenishing fluid loss. This of course will vary slightly according to the climate and the intensity of the exercise activity.

Water should be the most common fluid children consume throughout the day, as it replaces fluid loss and is the best choice for keeping their teeth healthy. So long as they are not too high in sugar, other fluids such as flavoured milk, fruit juices and cordial can be interspersed between drinks of water as they still keep children hydrated and have additional benefits such as the calcium in milk and the vitamin C in juices. Fruits such as watermelon also have a high water content, which helps keep children hydrated.

NUTRITION PRIOR TO AND DURING EXERCISE

Pre-exercise nutrition

If a child is scheduled to exercise in the morning, it is important they consume at least a small amount of food or drink with carbohydrate in it before they start. The purpose is to replace the essential blood glycogen stores in the liver, which become depleted overnight. Stores of glycogen in the brain are not high and if the liver stores are also low when a child commences exercising, then they may not receive enough glycogen to the brain, resulting in distraction and lethargy. Children can have a banana, a jam sandwich, crumpets and honey or a similar snack. These are foods that will help supply the body with essential blood glucose after an evening of fasting. The serving sizes should not be too large—if a meal is too substantial, the majority of blood focuses on the digestive system rather than the working muscles when exercising. A banana or a light sandwich is sufficient about 1 or 2 hours prior to exercising. This is also relevant for training at other times of the day. The body needs about 3 or 4 hours to process large meals before exercising.

There are some foods children might need to avoid before exercise. Milk products (even the amount on cereal) could create stomach upsets, especially if running or performing high-intensity exercise. High-fat meals can take too long to digest and foods high in salt can cause dehydration. Consuming too much sugar prior to exercise can also create stomach cramps. Some children find food and fluids that are high in fructose, such as fruits and fruit juice, can cause them problems if consumed in moderate to high volumes before exercising. As with most things, children will vary in their reactions (Richards n.d.).

Being hydrated is important, but determining the amount that children should drink prior to exercising will need some experimentation with. Some children will need to go to the bathroom constantly if they consume too much fluid prior to events. If training in the morning, some children will get up and have a glass of water or juice, and then prefer to drink during training and consume a substantial amount of water or fluids after training.

Nutrition and hydration during exercise

Unless children are participating in exercise of more than 1 hour's duration, it will not be essential that they eat during the exercise session, however, if the sport has breaks during the session then small amounts of food can be consumed, especially those with high water content, such as a few pieces of orange or watermelon.

Unless the exercise duration is less than 15 or 20 minutes, it is very important for children to drink during the exercise period to avoid dehydration. Ensure children have access to fluids and are adequately hydrated. This is especially important if the children are exercising on a hot day, as children are more prone to heat-related problems than adults are.

Dehydration can cause fatigue and impair muscle endurance. As a coach, you can teach children to drink prior to, during and after training. You can explain to carers the methods of judging water hydration in children such as checking urine colour. You can also explain that children may drink more if the fluids are flavoured and cold, so allowing children these options just before (unless milk-based), during and after exercise can be an option (Rowland 2011). While milk products might cause stomach upsets during exercise, they are ideal for aiding recovery after exercising.

If the exercise runs throughout the entire day, small snacks are recommended. These should be taken consistently over the day to sustain a child's energy. Examples of small snacks suitable for in between exercise activities include bananas, jam sandwiches, jelly lollies and fluids such as water, sports drinks and cordial. At the end of the exercise day, a medium to large carbohydrate- and protein-based meal should be consumed to assist recovery.

NUTRITION TO AID RECOVERY

Non-nutritional elements such as stretching, cold-water immersion, compression and sports massage can assist children to recover from exercise. Good nutrition and fluid replacement also play an important role in enhancing recovery. During intense exercise and extreme heat, children can lose up to 2 litres of fluid in an hour, so replacing lost fluid is an important skill to teach children.

After children have finished exercising, it is recommended that they consume a small carbohydrate and protein snack within 30 minutes to promote recovery. Examples of these include: a cheese sandwich; a jam sandwich and a flavoured milk drink; an icy pole and an English muffin with peanut butter; yoghurt and cereal; or a sports drink. The purpose of the carbohydrate is to replace the blood glycogen stores used during exercise. This is particularly important if the child will be exercising again within 12 hours' time. The purpose of the protein is to increase muscle repair (Cox n.d.).

After exercising, the child's next proper meal should include a medium to high level of carbohydrate, depending on the duration of the exercise. If the exercise duration was over an hour then a high carbohydrate meal will be important to fully replace glycogen levels. Protein should also be included to aid in muscle tissue repair and recovery (Cox n.d.).

If children are exercising for a long duration they will also lose sodium through sweating. Lost sodium is generally replaced through normal eating patterns.

SPORTS DRINKS

Rowland (2011) explains that children may drink larger volumes of fluid if the fluid is flavoured and cold. Allowing children to drink sports drinks only before, during and after exercise may assist them in increasing their fluid intake, especially in hot weather and for sporting activities over 1 hour in duration.

Sports drinks have been specifically designed to increase the rate of fluid absorption into the body and to replace the sodium and carbohydrates lost. However, they have been designed for adult fluid absorption needs so this should be kept in mind. Some sports drinks designed for children are now coming onto the market.

You can offer children other fluids as an alternative to sports drinks. Icy poles, cordial and fruit juices are also helpful in replenishing and maintaining children's fluid levels. These do not contain the same sodium content of a sports drink but they have a higher level of carbohydrates and are especially handy after exercising. Be careful, though—prior to exercise, high-sugar fluids such as cordial may cause cramping, and the fructose in juice may cause discomfort in the stomach. Adding a small amount of cordial or fruit juice to a larger volume of water can help avoid this problem. Milk products may need to be avoided before and during exercise as these can cause stomach upsets, however, they are perfect for after exercise.

How sports drinks work

The benefits of sports drinks for children mainly centre on increasing fluid intake to reduce dehydration. Sports drinks have been designed to replace sodium and to provide an optimal level of carbohydrates for the adult body to replace muscle glycogen quickly. The sodium and carbohydrate benefits are greatest for exercise sessions of 1 hour or more in duration. Children do not normally train or compete for longer than an hour so consuming cold water with a small carbohydrate and protein snack within 30 minutes after exercising is usually sufficient. It is not necessary for children exercising for less than an hour to consume sports drinks.

If children are training or competing for more than an hour then the sodium in sports drinks can replace that lost through sweat and prompt the thirst mechanism to drink more. Sodium is the main electrolyte in sports drinks; the other is potassium, which is beneficial in helping muscle contraction during exercise. The main benefit of a sports drink is for a child exercising for over an hour, especially in endurance and high-intensity sports, to avoid dehydration and replace glycogen stores lost.

If giving or suggesting sports drinks to children, it is recommended that:

▶ where possible, they are designed for children. This way, the balance of carbohydrates and electrolytes will be more in line with children's needs
▶ they only consume these drinks before, during and immediately after exercising. Water should be the staple drink for children, with some milk-based drinks for calcium
▶ they drink water after the sports drink to minimise the acidity residue left on the teeth which can create tooth enamel erosion
▶ they are aware that, unlike water, these drinks have kilojoules and if consumed in too high a quantity, could contribute to weight gain
▶ they understand the drinks really hold the most benefit for sports conducted over an hour in duration (Burke & Cox 2010).

Overall, because sports drinks are cold and flavoured, children are more likely to drink these than water. However, there are other flavoured cold drinks children can be given as alternatives, which may be just as effective if the exercise is shorter than an hour in duration.

SUMMARY

▶ Carbohydrates are broken down in the body and stored as blood glycogen in the muscles and liver.

▶ Muscle stores of blood glycogen are limited and deplete after 60 to 90 minutes of exercise in adults. Research on children's depleting muscle blood glycogen stores has not yet been conducted.

▶ Generally, if children exercise for under 1 hour, they just need to focus on hydration and consuming adequate food after exercise to replace blood glycogen losses.

▶ Generally, if children exercise for over an hour then small carbohydrate-rich snacks and/or fluids should be consumed throughout the session to replace blood glycogen losses.

▶ Children should be hydrated before exercise and ensure they have an intake of fluid during training and afterwards to replace fluid lost.

▶ Testing for dehydration can include having them check whether their urine is clear in colour.

▶ If children are exercising in the morning, they should have a small snack to avoid 'brain drain', as blood glycogen stores in the liver deplete overnight.

▶ Medium to large meals should be avoided for 3 to 4 hours before exercising. A small snack can be consumed 1 to 2 hours prior to exercise.

▶ Children often prefer to drink cold and flavoured drinks so these may be used to increase fluid intake if necessary.

▶ Consuming a snack or fluid that is carbohydrate- and protein-rich within 30 minutes after exercising will promote recovery from exercise.

▶ Some products, such as milk, are not recommended prior to exercise as they can create stomach upsets, particularly in endurance and high-intensity events. Have these products after exercise instead.

REFLECTIVE QUESTIONS FOR THE COACH

- What is the duration of your training sessions and competitions? Do the children seem to be lacking in energy? Do you think this is due to dehydration, carbohydrate stores diminishing or the training being physically intense?
- If carers ask whether their child should be consuming sports drinks, how will you respond?
- What are the most important nutritional lessons you can teach carers and children in relation to exercise?
- What food and fluids would you recommend children have before, during and after exercise?
- What food and fluids should children avoid prior to and during exercise?
- How will you incorporate teaching these nutritional concepts? Can you get children to bring water bottles and have drink stops throughout the training session? Can you hold a nutritional talk night for carers?

CHAPTER SEVEN

CARING FOR AND PREVENTING INJURIES

One of your responsibilities as a coach is to create training sessions and environments that minimise injury risk. This chapter provides information on:

- coaching techniques which can reduce the risk of injury
- management of injuries sustained during training or competition
- common sporting injuries among children
- medical conditions for coaches to consider.

COACHING TECHNIQUES TO REDUCE INJURY RISK

Not every technique mentioned below will be practical for the sport you coach, but implementation of as many of these techniques as possible can help keep injuries to a minimum.

Matching a child's ability to the sporting level and activity

Placing an inexperienced child in a team with a far higher ability level than they can manage can be detrimental to the child's self-esteem and place the child and the other team members at risk of injury. There is a normal flow to sports and an inexperienced child is more likely to be in the wrong place at the wrong time and create a higher number of collisions. The child could also strain muscles from extensive use beyond what they can cope with. Try to match children with teams that are suited to their sporting ability.

Appreciating that contact sports have a higher risk of injury

While there can be injuries in non-contact sports, the likelihood of collision-related injuries increases in contact sports. Some children's sports have modified non-contact rules until children are older. If children are moving into a contact sport phase, you will need to prepare their training to cater for this introduction. Also, during training for contact sports, match children on height and weight rather than age, where possible, to minimise the risk of injury.

Modifying game rules for children

Reducing the field size so children are not running the entire distance of an adult field or modifying equipment, such as younger children in athletics using a plastic, smaller-sized javelin, can reduce the risk of sporting injuries. You should consider whether you could tailor your training and equipment to suit children's safety needs.

Teaching children how to warm up and cool down

An effective warm-up and cool-down can reduce the risk of injury from training. A warm-up should involve warming the body through light exercise followed by stretching. The stretching should also be light in intensity and then move to a more moderate intensity. The warm-up should be sufficient so that when the main component of the training session commences, the child's body is warm, stretched and prepared for activity. The warm-up routine should also involve muscles and activities that are predominately used in the sport being performed (Nieman 2007).

Clark (2010) explains that an inadequate warm-up and a large volume of pre-exercise food or fluids can contribute to stitches occurring. A stitch is a pain just above the abdomen area while exercising. To treat a stitch, try breathing deeply and bend over to touch the ground. Bending over stretches the area and breathing deeply produces more oxygen to transport throughout the body. It also helps relax the abdominal area. Eyestone (2000) also suggests tightening and contracting the abdominal muscles.

The cool-down should reduce the heart rate, followed by static stretching. A similar warm-up and cool-down during each training session can help children remember and feel confident in completing these activities should you not be present.

Recommending rest and recovery

As a coach, you will not have a great deal of influence in this area but promoting adequate rest and sleep is important. With adequate rest and sleep, children will recover from training more effectively and be less tired during training and competition, which in turn can help reduce the risk of injury.

In some prominent sporting events, sleeping before competition is difficult, due to stress the child may be experiencing. The anxiety-reducing techniques presented in Chapter 5 (see p. 76) will be useful to assist in the management of this.

Providing adequate protective gear and equipment

Providing protective sporting gear is a proactive way to prevent injuries. Ensure the club has the appropriate mandatory sporting gear and equipment for children and that it is regularly checked. If children need to wear protective gear, ensure they understand how to fit the equipment properly.

Some protective or preventative sporting gear is not mandatory but can assist in avoiding injuries and it is worth encouraging the investment, for example, a quality pair of running shoes that have the correct support.

Setting training periodisation

Training periodisation is where training is split into different phases. The phases cater for the beginning of a season, building up to the peak of competition and then a rest phase after competition. The benefits of training periodisation are that training gradually progresses in intensity, frequency and/or duration. If children start at a lower intensity they will be less likely to sustain injuries or experience muscle soreness. Muscle soreness usually occurs from exercise children are unaccustomed to. The aim is to gradually build these training factors.

Training periodisation normally has three phases: the preparatory phase, the competition phase and the transition phase.

Preparatory phase

This is the training phase designed for the start of the season. It consists of pre-season training and the early stages of competition. The training focus is on increasing children's fitness and skill levels. As time evolves, the training becomes more focused on preparing children to peak at the main competition stage of the sport. The focus will then be more on maintaining rather than increasing fitness, and there will be a greater concentration on sport-specific skill development.

A substantial number of injuries occur early in the training phase. This is when children have not yet developed their motor skills beyond the most basic level and their fitness may also be lacking. It is important to allow children the opportunity to develop their skills and fitness levels before placing them in competition or intense exercise environments. This will help minimise their risk of injury.

Competition phase

This training phase is not the entire competition season of the sport. Children are not able to maintain peak level over the entire season. This phase usually starts about four to six weeks prior to competition. Higher-intensity, shorter-duration fitness training is undertaken and there is a strong focus on skill development. Children should have a strong base from the preparatory phase to be able to endure the higher-intensity training without sustaining injuries. The week prior to competition, a reduction in training and more rest is incorporated to ensure that on competition day children are fully rested with no muscle soreness and their energy systems are fully recovered. The competition phase is short as children can only sustain high-intensity training for a short period of time before reaching the overtraining stage, which results in reduced performance and higher risk of injury. The immune system is also affected by overtraining and children will be more susceptible to colds and flu.

Transition phase

When the competition finishes, children have a recovery and rest period. Many children participate in a variety of sports over different seasons so they may finish one sport and move straight on to the next. It is recommended that after a period of intense competition children have light training for about four weeks.

Evaluating the training surface

The type of surface children train and compete on can have an influence on the probability of their sustaining an injury. If children are training on a hard surface, occasionally arrange for them to train on grass or hold a beach session on the sand. Hard surfaces can place more stress on the body, particularly for weight-bearing exercise, and place children at more risk of sustaining an injury.

In sports like yachting and outdoor cycling, the environment—such as rain or windy weather—can put children at greater risk of sustaining an injury. Each sport needs to be evaluated and coaching instructions modified depending on environmental conditions. For example, if children are playing a netball game in the rain, you can give instructions to make shorter passes and play a slower, steadier game.

Uneven or sloped playing fields or those with potholes need to be avoided where possible. Mixed spaces, such as in athletics where numerous events are occurring at the same time, can create a higher risk of injury too. If you are coaching your athletes on a field with other sports or groups of people training, you will need to create an environment and instructions that assist in improving safety and work with these other groups to define boundaries.

Discovering the major injuries for the sport

Harris and Anderson (2010) explain that the more knowledgeable and experienced a coach is, the less likely it is that injuries will occur.

Completing research into any injuries that occur in your sport can help you design a stretching and strength program to strengthen the muscles in and around the areas of likely injury. For example, if knee injuries are common in your sport you can design a warm-up that stretches and strengthens the quadriceps, hamstrings and iliotibial band, and brainstorm ideas that could lead to prevention at training and in competition.

Once a child has sustained an injury, it is more likely that this area could be re-injured. Prevention is always the best option, but once a child has sustained an injury and it has healed it is still important to ensure the child has a stretching and strength program tailored specifically to strengthen the previously injured area.

Minimising the risk of heat illness

Children do not have the same cooling efficiency as adults and are more susceptible to heat illness. You will need to be aware of this and ensure children drink plenty of fluids, and where possible train and hold events in the cooler parts of the day.

Appreciating that certain children are natural risk-takers

Children are likely to be less informed about the risks of certain situations or may prefer more injury-prone sports such as snowboarding, football, surfing and diving. For these sports it is very important that a knowledgeable coach is instructing the children. Both you, as the coach, and the child's carers are responsible for instructing children about how to keep as safe as possible during training and competition. These sports also have build-up phases and it is important the children work through the phases. In diving, for example, there are different platform heights and differences in difficulty of dives performed. For safety, a child should start with the basics and progress through the levels of difficulty.

Recognising that a child may disguise an injury

Children like to please their carers and coaches so they may disguise an injury to continue participating in a sport. It is important you convey the message that if a child experiences any pain or is injured that you are to be informed. Make it clear that the child will not get in trouble, you will not be upset with them and they will not be letting the team down. If you are told, then you can take steps to help make the injury better. If a child continues exercising with an injury it can become worse and may take longer to heal.

MANAGEMENT OF INJURIES

During your coaching sessions, it is highly likely you will experience one of the children sustaining an injury so it is important to have at least a basic understanding of injury management.

Non-life-threatening injuries

Thankfully, most injuries children sustain will be mild contusions (bruises), sprains and strains. This section explains what to do in the event a child sustains a non-life-threatening injury. The injury management approach is explained through the acronym RICER, which stands for rest, ice, compression, elevation, referral (St John Ambulance 2006).

Rest

If a child is injured, ask them to stop participating in the training session or competition and let you assess the level of injury before allowing them to resume exercise. The aim is to avoid further injury. If it is likely the child will be causing further damage to the injury if they continue, they should no longer participate in that training session or competition.

Ice

Place an icepack (or similar) within a wet cloth onto the injured area. Keep this on the injury for 15 minutes and explain to the child's carer to repeat the process every 2 hours for the first day. During the next day, the injured area should be iced for 15 minutes every 4 hours. During the first 48 hours it is best to avoid heat and massage on the injury to minimise swelling and bleeding.

Compression

Place a compression bandage or something similar around and just above and below the injured area. Wrap the bandage around the area in a firm manner to stop extra blood flow and fluid formation, which will help reduce the swelling that could occur. Make sure the compression bandage is not so tight that it restricts the blood flow. You can check this by judging the colour of the skin under the bandage. Make sure the colour is the same as outside the bandaged area. If it is slightly blue or paler, the bandage is too tight.

Some children will wear a bandage as a form of compression until the injury has fully recovered, to provide additional physical and in some cases emotional support.

Elevation

Elevate the injured area. If the child has injured their calf then ideally they will lie down and have their leg propped up on a pillow while it is being iced and for the rest of the day. The purpose of raising the injured area is to reduce swelling and blood flow to the injury.

Referral

In some cases, the child will need to see a doctor or physiotherapist to properly diagnose and treat the injury. The next section explains when to do this. If these RICER measures are taken then hopefully the pain should be reduced over a 24- to 48-hour period, and if the child can exercise pain-free, they can resume training.

Referral to a doctor or physiotherapist

Harris and Anderson (2010) suggest referring a child to a doctor, hospital or physiotherapist if the child:

▶   says they are experiencing severe pain

▶ seems to have a joint injury such as a dislocation or the joint is very unstable

▶ has lost movement, for example, they are unable to walk because of a twisted ankle or injured knee

▶ initially seems to have suffered a minor injury yet it has not healed within two weeks

▶ seems to have an injury which has become infected.

Medical decisions reside with the child's caregiver, however, if you are at all concerned about the nature of an injury, it is always important that you suggest the child is referred to a professional for medical treatment and to follow up. Build up your network of contacts so that you can recommend some suitable doctors to carers. If medical treatment is not sought, then injuries can worsen and potentially mean children are unable to exercise for long periods of time.

Recovering from a non-life-threatening injury

A common question is how long children need to rest for before they can return to sport after injury. If the child has been referred to a doctor, physiotherapist or similar specialist then the carer and coach will be advised of a time frame. This is normally based on the type and severity of the injury. Generally, a child can return to exercise if they can stretch and exercise the injured part with no pain. Most doctors and physiotherapists will recommend stretches and strengthening exercises to assist the child's ability to return to sport and prevent re-injury.

Life-threatening injuries

For the management of serious injuries, time is crucial. It is highly recommended that you complete a first-aid course.

If a child experiences a life-threatening injury, you should follow the procedures known as DR ABCD, which stands for danger, response, airway, breathing, compression, defibrillation (St John Ambulance 2006).

Danger

Check before approaching the child that you are not putting yourself or others in danger. This is more critical in situations such as car crashes and electrical accidents, however, it is still always a first point of observation.

Response

When it is safe to approach the child, approach them and call their name and lightly shake them on the shoulder. The aim is to determine if you receive a response from the child. If there is a response and the child is injured, then you need to assess whether to get them immediately to a doctor or follow the RICER procedure. If there is no response then you need to request that someone immediately calls an ambulance.

Airway

If no response is given, roll the child onto their side into the coma (recovery) position. Sometimes a child is already lying on their side so you can keep them there and make small adjustments to achieve the coma position. The main purpose is to ensure their airway is clear. This book does not cover the details of how to move a child into a coma position. It is highly recommended that you complete a first-aid course or research this information further.

Breathing

If the child is breathing but not moving, keep them in the coma position until the ambulance arrives. Continuously check their breathing.

Compression

In the case of life-threating injuries when the child is not breathing, cardiopulmonary resuscitation (CPR) needs to be performed.

If the child is not breathing, you will need to immediately roll the child from the coma position onto their back. You will need to give the child two initial breaths by tilting their head back and pinching their nose to stop the air escaping. If there is no sign of life and no breathing then commence compressions on their chest. To do this, place your two hands together, palms down. The palms of your hands should be placed on the middle of the sternum area and pressed down about 4 or 5 centimetres, giving 30 compressions followed by 2 breaths for 5 sets, which should take about 2 minutes. You continue this until the child responds by starting to breathe, the ambulance arrives or a more experienced practitioner such as a doctor takes over.

Defibrillation

Defibrillation is a recent addition to this acronym. It is now recommended that defibrillation devices are included in first-aid kits. The devices contain verbal instructions on how to apply them to a child in a life-threatening situation such as when the child is unconscious and not breathing.

In any of these stages, never give a child food or drink if you suspect they have a serious injury.

COMMON SPORTING INJURIES

In Australia, increasing numbers of children are becoming involved in organised sport, and there has been a subsequent increase in sporting injuries among children. This does not mean children should stop participating in competitive sport—it offers many benefits such as social interaction, increased fitness, motor skill development and increased self-esteem. It does mean that you should be aware of proper injury management and methods to reduce the risk of injuries occurring.

Contact sports and sports that involve jumping, such as volleyball, usually create more injuries. The most common sporting injuries are mild contusions, sprains and strains. After this, the upper extremities such as the hands, followed by the lower extremities such as the legs are common locations of injuries in children participating in sport. A small percentage of children receive head injuries. When children grow older they are more likely to experience injuries to their lower extremities as opposed to their upper extremities. About one in 10 injuries will involve a fracture.

Overall, youth sports are considered relatively safe. Injury rates do increase as children become older. Boys are more likely to sustain injuries than girls are, and they are more likely to be of greater severity.

Types of injuries
Injuries can be classified in the following ways:

▶ trauma injuries, which are those that involve contact in a sport, such as running into an opponent on the football field
▶ muscular injuries, which are those that occur to muscles, tendons, joints or ligaments, such as pulling a hamstring when kicking a goal in football
▶ overuse injuries, which involve the continual strain on muscles, joints, tendons or bones, causing the area to become painful.

Trauma and muscular injuries differ to overuse injuries in that they are normally caused by a sudden stress. Trauma and muscular injuries normally deliver a sudden, sharp pain straightaway. In runners, if sprinting, muscular injuries will normally occur in the hamstring, thigh and occasionally the calf muscle.

Overuse injuries account for about one-third of all reported injuries. These occur when the child consistently puts strain on a particular area, and are common in children who are training at high intensity, frequency and duration. Long-distance runners are prone to overuse injuries in the hamstring, calf, Achilles tendon and iliotibial band. For throwers, injuries occur both in the legs and the upper arms. Overuse injuries can feel like a dull pain getting worse the longer training and competition goes on, or the pain can come on suddenly like trauma and muscular pain.

Each of these injury types will need to be managed using the RICER approach.

If children participate in sporting activities they are not accustomed to, they may experience muscle soreness. Muscle soreness can remain for up to three days after exercise. It can be treated using the RICER approach, and gentle stretching and warm baths can also assist with pain management. If pain persists after three days then there is a possibility that the child has sustained an injury.

Levels of overuse injuries

Overuse injuries can be classified in levels to help explain how serious the injury is and the likely recovery duration.

Level 1

This is the lowest level of injury occurrence. A child will normally complain of a slight ache during exercise. The pain may continue for a short time after the exercise but then stop. At this stage it is important to apply the RICER procedures and give the child time off exercising until they can resume stretching and exercising pain-free. Refer to page 105 to determine whether the child should see a doctor or physiotherapist. Usually, though, with a low-level injury, a few days off and applying ice, compression and elevation should be sufficient to aid recovery.

The child may also be able to cross-train during this period. This means the child can still participate in exercise that does not place strain on the injured area. For example, if the child mildly injured their ankle running, then swimming and cycling are cross-training options as they place less body weight on the injured ankle area than running does; if a shoulder is injured then leg exercises such as squats can still be performed.

Level 2

This is the level when pain from an injury occurs during the exercise activity and the child needs to stop, as the pain is too great for them to continue training. The pain also normally continues after the exercise has ceased, which is not usually the case in Level 1 injuries. In this instance, the injury is more severe and the RICER process will need to be immediately applied. The child will probably need time off sport and referral to a specialist. A physiotherapist will be able to advise what caused the problem if this is not known, what needs to be done to heal the injury and how much time the child will need to take off the sport. Time is a great healer of injuries so time off the sport and activity is important. It is also important to determine what created this level of pain. If the training level was too high then this will need to be amended to avoid the injury happening again, or maybe a strengthening exercise program needs to be developed for muscles and joints around the injured area. Once again, cross-training, such as training in the pool, can be incorporated to maintain fitness levels.

Level 3

This level involves significant pain to an injured area during and after exercise as with Level 2. The difference is that at Level 2, sometimes the child can start exercising again for a short period of time before having to stop. At Level 3 the child will be in immediate strong pain when trying to exercise. At this level the sporting activity may need to be suspended for six to eight weeks. Referral to a doctor or physiotherapist is usually needed. It is important that pain experienced by the child is immediately treated and the child is given rest from the exercise until they are fully recovered. Pushing a child injured at this level can create such a serious injury that they will require substantial time off the sport. In some cases, the child can return to a different sport while the injury heals. For example, a child may not be able to run due to an Achilles injury but they may be able to swim and complete some light cycling.

Level 4

This is the most severe level of injury. At this stage, the child is unable to perform for an extended period because of persistent pain at the injured area. Rest will need to occur for several months or the child may need to change sports. It can be very distressing for an athlete, child or adult, to sustain an injury this debilitating. Encouragement, specialised rehabilitation exercises and, where possible, participation in activities that do not put pressure on the injured part can help keep the child motivated and active.

The psychological impact of injuries

Sustaining an injury can be emotionally upsetting and frustrating for a child. They will no longer be able to participate in the sport they enjoy, or train and play with their team or friends. The concern is that the child will continue to exercise and make the injury worse or return too early. Offering cross-training options that do not aggravate the injury can assist in helping children remain in sport during the recovery phase.

Children can experience feelings of:

▶ nervousness about their competency level when they return
▶ concern about re-injury
▶ loneliness from not mixing with their friends and teammates
▶ concern about how long the injury may take to heal.

It is recommended that you arrange a progressive plan for the child when they return to training. This can help the child feel more confident about being able to train after time off and will allow for loss of fitness and strength in the injured area. It is a good idea to implement a specialised stretching and strength program for the injured area to minimise the chance of re-injury.

You will also need to set realistic short-term goals given the time off and injury. Explain to the child you do not expect them to be at the same level as when they became injured. When the child returns, arrange for them to participate in a lighter version of the game such as playing half the game or playing a full game for a lower grade before having the full pressure of a high-level match when not fully fit. In addition, invite the child to participate in any social events or assistant roles such as scoring at weekend competitions. This can help the child still feel part of the team.

MEDICAL CONDITIONS TO CONSIDER

There are medical conditions common in children which you will need to be informed about. Two of the more common conditions include asthma and diabetes. A brief section on children exercising with a cold is also discussed here.

Asthma

If a child suffers from asthma they can have trouble breathing, caused by a narrowing of their airways. Exercise can trigger an onset of asthma due to loss of heat and water from the child's airway passages. This is called exercise-induced asthma. Asthma is more common in continuous exercise than in start-stop sports such as netball and football. When asthma occurs it can range from mild breathing difficulty and coughing to serious breathing problems.

The way to treat asthma is to sit the child upright and reassure them, trying to keep the child as calm as possible. In most cases, the child will be aware they have asthma and will have a reliever inhaler with them or nearby. Help the child administer the reliever inhaler, giving them the number of puffs indicated on the inhaler. Wait for 4 minutes to see if their breathing improves. If there is no improvement in the situation, help the child administer another round of puffs. If no improvement is observed after this, call for an ambulance. If the child becomes unconscious, follow the DR ABCD protocol outlined in the earlier section of this chapter on life-threatening injuries (see p. 106).

When coaching a child with asthma, ensure they complete a sufficient warm-up to prepare their body for the main component of the training or competition session. This will help reduce their risk of experiencing exercise-induced asthma. You should also ensure that the child has their medication with them in easy access at all times. Having asthma should not preclude a child from participating in exercise, as exercise can be beneficial in reducing the number and severity of asthma occurrences.

Diabetes

If a child has diabetes this means their body is not able to produce enough insulin to regulate their blood sugar levels. Having diabetes should not preclude children from participating in exercise. Regular exercise has been found to help children maintain a steadier blood sugar level.

Children mostly fall into the category of type 1 diabetes. This typically occurs in people under the age of 30. It requires the child to replace insulin in their body through an injection, pen or pump.

Children with diabetes can experience low blood sugar during exercise, which is termed hypoglycaemia. If this occurs then medical attention will need to be sought. The onset of hypoglycaemia is very quick. A child will start to feel shaky, dizzy, anxious and disoriented. At this stage give the child some food or fluids with fast-acting sugar content such as fruit juice, sports drinks or lollies. The child should immediately feel better after this. It is also a good idea to follow this up with high-carbohydrate food. If a child becomes hypoglycaemic and is not treated immediately, they can become unconscious. No food or drink should be administered at this stage and DR ABCD steps need to be taken.

It is a highly recommended that you ask carers of children participating in your sport to complete a health questionnaire so that you have an understanding of any medical conditions.

Colds

Children often experience colds; the question is whether to let them train or compete in these situations. If the cold is mild and the child feels well enough to train then the child can train at a low intensity. They will need to have substantial rest and fluid intake after the training session. If a child is experiencing a cold at a medium to severe level then the child should rest until the cold has dissipated. In addition, if the child is taking any medication such as antibiotics then the child should not exercise regardless of how they feel or the cold intensity (mild to severe) until the course of the medication is completed or they are given advice from a medical practitioner to the contrary.

SUMMARY

▶ You can apply techniques such as evaluating the training terrain, modifying game rules, setting training periodisation and researching common injuries to reduce the injury risk for the children you coach.

▶ To manage non-life-threatening injuries, you should follow the RICER approach, which involves rest, ice, compression, elevation and referral.

▶ It is recommended you complete a first-aid course.

▶ Children can sustain three types of injuries: trauma, muscular and overuse injuries.

▶ Muscle soreness can occur when children participate in exercise their body is unaccustomed to. Muscle soreness can last around three days. If it lasts longer, the muscle may be injured and require expert treatment.

▶ Overuse injuries are classified into four levels depending on the severity of injury. The severity will influence when the child can return to exercise.

▶ Cross-training, such as training in a pool, can be an effective way for children to keep training while injured.

▶ If a child is returning from injury, a progressive training program should be devised and ideally the child should have a stretching and strength program for the area that was injured to reduce the risk of re-injury.

REFLECTIVE QUESTIONS FOR THE COACH

✎ Reflect on any injury you have had to treat. What type of injury was it? Was it a trauma, an overuse or a muscular injury? Was the injury avoidable? Was the RICER approach followed?

- Is there a common pattern of injuries in your sport? Does training intensity need to be amended or does a stretching and strengthening program for these types of injuries need to be added?
- What coaching techniques to reduce injury do you think you could implement at your training sessions? Could you research the major injuries of your sport and the best stretching and strength exercises to proactively reduce the risk of these injuries?
- Do you have a first-aid kit at training? Have you completed a first-aid course?
- What is the training environment like from an injury and safety point of view? For example, is the ground uneven? Are other groups training on the oval?
- Do you have a physiotherapist or sports doctor you can refer injured children to?
- Are there legalities surrounding your injury management responsibilities in your insurance policy? Do you have carers fill out a health questionnaire about their children? Do you have to report and refer all injuries?
- What would you do if a carer told you their child had a cold and they were not sure whether the child should train?
- What suggestions would you make to a child who experienced muscle soreness from the training session? Do you think you would need to modify training because of this?
- If a child sustains an injury, what kind of health professionals would you refer the child to? What suggestions for exercise programs would you make for assisting with recovery in conjunction with or supporting any medical rehabilitation program the child might be prescribed, such as gentle stretching or water-based rehabilitation exercises? If a child were feeling upset because they sustained an injury, what would you say to them?
- How would you determine if a child should keep training if they seemed in pain? Have you spoken to the children about talking to you if they experience pain or an injury?

MORE INFORMATION

Australian Council for Health, Physical Education and Recreation
www.achper.org.au/
Australian Sports Commission—Coaching and Officiating Development home page
www.ausport.gov.au/participating/coachofficial
Australian Sports Commission—*Sports Coach* online magazine
www.ausport.gov.au/sportscoachmag/home
Australian Strength and Conditioning Association
www.strengthandconditioning.org/
National Sporting Organisation contacts—Australian sports directory
www.ausport.gov.au/about/australian_sport_directory
Sports Medicine Australia
www.sma.org.au/
Sports Science Education Institute
www.sportsscienceeducation.com.au
State Department of Sport and Recreation coaching contacts
www.ausport.gov.au/participating/coaches/further_information

Sporting coaches associations such as:

Australian Tennis Professional Coaches Association
www.atpca.com.au/
Australian Track and Field Coaches Association
www.atfca.com.au/
Basketball Australia
www.basketball.net.au/index.php?id=347
Cricket Australia
www.cricket.com.au/get-involved/coaching
Football Federation Australia
www.footballaustralia.com.au/getinvolved/coaching
Gymnastics Australia
www.gymnastics.org.au/default.asp?MenuID=Coaching_@_Judging/
c20038/3023
Hockey Australia
www.hockey.org.au/Participate/Coaching
Netball Australia
www.netball.asn.au/extra.asp?id=16023&OrgID=1&menu=10664
Rowing Australia
www.rowingaustralia.com.au/dev_coaches.shtm
SwimEd
www.swimed.com/swimming-coaching

GLOSSARY

Aerobic training is exercise conducted at a level where sufficient amounts of oxygen are being transported to the heart and working muscles to sustain the activity.

Anaerobic training is exercise that exceeds the body's ability to transport blood and oxygen to the heart and working muscles, resulting in a build-up of lactic acid.

Ballistic stretching is stretching where a bouncing motion occurs at the peak of the stretch.

Biological age is the age of a child in terms of their physical maturity.

Circuit training involves completing a set number of different exercises at different stations over an allocated period of time.

Closed motor skills are those conducted when the target or object is stationary and the environment is stable.

Developmental age is a combination of a child's physical maturity and their emotional and social development.

Discrete motor skills are those that have a definite start and finish.

Dynamic stretches are performed in a slow, steady motion throughout the exercise.

Extrinsic motivation is the drive to complete activities because of external rewards.

Fartlek training involves exercise completed for a short period of time at medium to high intensity followed by exercise at a lower intensity. This process is then repeated.

Fine motor skills involve a small number of muscles used to create movement, such when writing.

Gross motor skills involve large muscle groups within the body to create movement, such as when running.

Growth plates are located at the end of a child's long bones and are made up of growing tissue.

Interval training involves exercise completed for a short period of time at medium to high intensity followed by a rest period. This process is then repeated.

Intrinsic motivation is the drive to complete activities for personal reasons.

Lactic acid is a by-product resulting from anaerobic exercise.

Motor skills are voluntary, learnt movements made by the human body to achieve a task, such as moving the arm to throw a tennis ball.

Open motor skills are those conducted when the target or object is in motion and the environment is changing.

Overtraining occurs when a child is exposed to training at too high an intensity, duration or frequency, resulting in reduced performance, increased tiredness, increased risk of injury and reduced immune function, along with other symptoms.

Plyometric training is exercise that creates a contraction then relaxation of the muscle and usually involves jumping-type activities such as skipping.

Progressive overload is a gradual increase in the frequency, intensity or duration of exercise to create improvement.

Progressive muscular relaxation is a technique that involves relaxing major muscle groups of the body one at a time.

Proprioceptive neuromuscular facilitation (PNF) stretching involves a stretch against resistance to create muscle contraction.

Reversibility is when training ceases and a loss in physical adaptations and in some cases motor skill development can occur; also known as detraining.

Serial motor skills are discrete motor skills completed in a series.

Simplification of practice applies techniques to make a skill easier to perform.

Specificity of practice is practice of the exact actions and exercise activities that will enhance development within that specific sport.

Static stretches are stretches held in one position for around 30 seconds.

Thermal stress refers to the negative impact of extreme temperatures on a child's body.

Training age is the number of years a child has participated in a sport.

Training periodisation is a training plan that has different objectives over a period of time in sync with the sporting season, such as a preparatory and competition phase.

Transtheoretical model relates to the readiness of a person to participate in an activity.

Variability of practice involves training sessions that have changing elements, such as the difficulty of the skills or changing terrain, to improve motor skill adaptability.

Visualisation is a technique using mind imagery to increase confidence and reinforce positive practice.

REFERENCES

American Academy of Orthopaedic Surgeons 2010, 'Growth plate fractures', *OrthoInfo: your connection to expert orthopaedic information*, http://orthoinfo. aaos.org/topic.cfm?topic=A00040

Anderson, B 2000, *Stretching*, Shelter Publications, California.

Anshel, M 2011, *Sport psychology from theory to practice*, 5th edn, Benjamin Cummings, San Francisco.

Australian Bureau of Statistics 2011, *Obesity*, www.abs.gov.au/ausstats/abs@.nsf/ Lookup/by%20Subject/1370.0~2010~Chapter~Obesity%20(4.1.6.6.3)

Australian Sports Commission (n.d. a), 'Sporting attire', *Participating in sport*, Australian Government, Canberra, www.ausport.gov.au/participating/ women/resources/issues/attire

Australian Sports Commission (n.d. b), 'Weight training for young athletes', *Participating in sport*, Australian Government, Canberra, www.ausport.gov. au/participating/coaches/tools/coaching_children/Weight_training

Australian Sports Commission 2008, *Coaching children*, Australian Government, Canberra, www.ausport.gov.au/__data/assets/pdf_file/0017/380231/ SP_32434_Coaching_Children.pdf

Australian Strength and Conditioning Association 2007, *Resistance training for children and youth: a position stand from the Australian Strength and Conditioning Association*, ASCA, Beenleigh, www.strengthandconditioning.org/images/ PositionStand/asca%20position%20stand%20resistance%20training%20 for%20children%20and%20youth%20nov%202007%20-%20final.pdf

Bailey, R, Morley, D & Dismore, H 2009, 'Talent development in physical education: a national survey of policy and practice in England', *Physical Education & Sport Pedagogy*, vol. 14, no. 1, pp. 59–73.

Baker, J, Cobley, S & Thomas, J 2009, 'What do we know about early sport specialization? Not much!', *High Ability Studies*, vol. 20, no. 1, pp. 77–89.

Balyi, I & Hamilton, A 2003, 'Long-term athlete development update: trainability in childhood and adolescence', *Faster, Higher, Stronger*, vol. 20, pp. 6–8.

Beihoff, C & Pop, M 2009, 'Strength training for children and adolescents: is it beneficial?', *Science, Movement and Health*, no. 1, pp. 12–14.

Boreham, C & McKay, H 2011, 'Physical activity in childhood and bone health', *British Journal of Sports Medicine*, vol. 45, pp. 877–9.

Burke, L & Cox, G 2010, *The complete guide to food for sports performance*, 3rd edn, Allen & Unwin, Sydney.

Burke, L & Deakin, V 2008, *Clinical sports nutrition*, 3rd edn, The McGraw Companies, Sydney.

Caine, D, DiFiori, J & Maffuli, N 2006, 'Physical injuries in children and youth sports: reason for concern?', *British Journal of Sports Medicine*, vol. 40, no. 9, pp. 749–61.

Capranica, L & Millard-Stafford, M 2011, 'Youth sport specialization: how to manage competition and training?', *International Journal of Sports Physiology & Performance*, vol. 6, no. 4, pp. 572–80.

Clark, N 2010, 'Undesired sideliners: side stitches and runner's trots', *Running & FitNews*, vol. 28, no. 4, July–August.

Clements, M (n.d.) 'How to get your group to become a team', *Sports Coach*, vol. 29, no. 2.

Commonwealth Scientific Industrial Research Organisation 2008, *2007 Australian national children's nutrition and physical activity survey: main findings*, Department of Health and Ageing, Commonwealth of Australia, Canberra, www.health.gov.au/internet/main/publishing.nsf/content/66596E8FC68FD1A3CA2574D50027DB86/$File/childrens-nut-phys-survey.pdf

Cox, G (n.d.), 'Nutritional strategies to maximise recovery following strenuous exercise', *Sports Coach*, vol. 28, no. 4.

Crespo, M & McInerney, P 2006, 'Talent identification and development in tennis', *Coaching and Sports Science Review*, vol. 39, pp. 2–4.

Cross, N & Lyle, J (eds) 1999, *The coaching process: principles and practice for sport*, Butterworth-Heinemann, Oxford.

CSIRO, see Commonwealth Sciencific Industrial Research Organisation

Davey, M 2012, 'Can't run, can't throw: motor skills wide of the mark', *Sydney Morning Herald*, 24 July, www.smh.com.au/national/health/cant-run-cant-throw--motor-skills-wide-of-the-mark-20120723-22koo.html

Department of Health and Ageing 2004a, *Australia's physical activity recommendations for 5–12 year olds*, Australian Government, Canberra, www.health.gov.au/internet/main/publishing.nsf/content/phd-physical-activity-kids-pdf-cnt.htm

Department of Health and Ageing 2004b, *Australia's physical activity recommendations for 12–18 year olds*, Australian Government, Canberra, www.health.gov.au/internet/main/publishing.nsf/content/phd-physical-activity-youth-pdf-cnt.htm

Department of Sport and Recreation 2003, *Keep it fun: supporting youth sport. Clubs guide to encouraging positive parent behaviour*, Government of Western Australia, Wembley, fulltext.ausport.gov.au/fulltext/2003/wa/keepitfun.pdf

Egger, G & Champion, N (eds) 1998, *The fitness leader's handbook*, 4th edn, Kangaroo Press, Kenthurst, New South Wales.

Eyestone, E 2000, 'Remove your stitches', *Runner's World*, vol. 35, no. 12, p. 40.

Faigenbaum, AD & Chu, DA 2007, *Plyometric training for children and adults*, American College of Sports Medicine, Indianapolis, Indiana, www.acsm.org/docs/current-comments/plyometrictraining.pdf

Faigenbaum, AD, Kraemer, WJ, Blimkie, CJR, Jeffreys, I, Micheli, LJ, Nitka, M & Rowland, TW, 2009, 'Youth resistance training: updated position statement paper from the National Strength and Conditioning Association', *Journal of Strength & Conditioning Research*, vol. 23, S60–79.

Fitts, PM & Posner, MI 1967, *Human performance*, Brooks/Cole, Belmont, California.

Fleming, N & Baume, D 2006, 'Learning styles again: VARKing up the right tree!', *Educational Developments*, vol. 7, no. 4, pp. 4–7.

Gearity, B 2012, 'Poor teaching by the coach: a phenomenological description from athletes' experience of poor coaching', *Routledge Physical Education and Sport Pedagogy*, vol. 17, no. 1, pp. 79–96.

Gerrard, D 1993, 'Overuse injuries and growing bones: the young athlete at risk', *British Journal of Sports Medicine*, vol. 27, no. 1, pp. 14–18.

Glover, B & Glover, S 1999, *The competitive runner's handbook*, Penguin Books, New York.

Gould, D, Chung, Y, Smith, P & White, J 2006, 'Future directions in coaching life skills: understanding high school coaches' views and needs', *Athletic Insight: the online journal of sports psychology*, vol. 8, no. 3, www.athleticinsight.com/Vol8Iss3/CoachingPDF.pdf

Gould, D, Lauer, L, Rolo, C, Jannes, C & Pennisi, NS, 2006, 'Understanding the role parents play in tennis success: a national survey of junior tennis coaches', *British Journal of Sports Medicine*, vol. 40, no. 7, pp. 632–6.

Granacher, U, Roggo, K, Wischer, T, Fischer, S, Zuerny, C, Gollhofer, A & Kriemler, S 2011, 'Effects and mechanisms of strength training in children', *International Journal of Sports Medicine*, vol. 32, no. 5, pp. 357–65.

Halls, M. (n.d.) 'The challenge of engaging young children in sport', *Sports Coach*, vol. 28, no. 4, Australian Sports Commission, Camberra, www.ausport.gov.au/sportscoachmag/coaching_processes/the_challenge_of_engaging_young_children_in_sport

Harris, S & Anderson, S 2010, *Care of the young athlete*, 2nd edn, American Academy of Pediatrics, Elk Grove Village, Illinois.

Hedstrom, R, & Gould, D 2004, *Research in youth sports: critical issues status*, Institute for the Study of Youth Sports, Michigan State University, East Lansing.

Heyward, V 2010, *Advanced fitness assessment and exercise prescription*, 6th edn, Human Kinetics, Champaign, Illinois.

Hill, B & Green, C 2008, 'Give the bench the boot! Using manning theory to design youth sport programs', *Journal of Sport Management*, vol. 22, pp. 184–204.

Howley, E & Franks, D 2007, *Fitness professional's handbook*, 5th edn, Human Kinetics, Champaign, Illinois.

Humphrey, J 2003, *Child development through sports*, Haworth Press, New York.

Johnson, B, Salzberg, C & Stevenson, D 2011, 'Systematic review: plyometric training programs for young children', *Journal of Strength & Conditioning Research*, vol. 25, no. 9, pp. 2623–34.

Lavay, B, Henderson, H, French, R & Guthrie, S 2011, 'Behavior management instructional practices and content of college/university physical education teacher education (PETE) programs', *Physical Education and Sport Pedagogy*, vol. 17, no. 2, pp. 195–210.

Magill, R 2007, *Motor learning and control concepts and applications*, 8th edn, McGraw-Hill, New York.

McFarland, AL 2011, 'Growing minds: the relationship between parental attitude about nature and the development of fine and gross motor skills in children', PhD thesis, Texas A&M University, College Station.

McMorris, T 2004, *Acquisition and performance of sports skills*, John Wiley and Sons, Oxford.

Moesch, K, Elbe, A, Hause, M & Wikman, J 2011, 'Late specialization: the key to success in centimeters, grams, or seconds (cgs) sports', *Scandinavian Journal of Medicine & Science in Sports*, vol. 21, no. 6, pp. 282–91.

Nieman, D 2007, *Exercise testing and prescription*, 6th edn, McGraw Hill, New York.

Noakes, T 2003, *Lore of running*, 4th edn, Human Kinetics, Champaign, Illinois.

Pangrazi, R 2007, *Dynamic physical education for elementary school children*, 15th edn, Pearson, San Francisco.

Patel, D, Pratt, H & Greydanus, D 2002, 'Pediatric neurodevelopment and sports participation: when are children ready to play sports?', *Pediatric Clinics of North America*, vol. 49, no. 3, pp. 505–31.

Ratel, S, Duche, P & Williams, S 2006, 'Muscle fatigue during high-intensity exercise in children', *Sports Medicine*, vol. 36, no. 12, pp. 1031–65.

Ratel, S, Lazaar, N, Dore, E & Baquet, G 2004, 'High-intensity intermittent activities at school: controversies and facts', *Journal of Sports Medicine and Physical Fitness*, vol. 44. no. 3, pp. 272–80.

Richards, C (n.d.), 'When good food bites you back: understanding food allergy and intolerance', *Sports Coach*, vol. 27, no. 3.

Rink, J 2002, *Teaching physical education for learning*, 6th edn, McGraw Higher Education, New York.

Rowland, T 2002, 'Exercise physiology: are children unique?', paper presented at the Australian Conference of Science and Medicine in Sport 2002: Sports medicine and science at the extremes, Melbourne, 12–16 October.

Rowland, T 2011, 'Fluid replacement requirements for child athletes', *Sports Medicine*, vol. 41, no. 4, p. 279.

Shaw, D, Gorely, T & Corban, R 2005, *Sport and exercise psychology*, Garland Science/BIOS Scientific Publications, Abingdon, Oxfordshire.

Sibte, N 2003, *Weight training—pre-adolescent strength training—just do it!*, www.ausport.gov.au/participating/coaches/tools/coaching_children/Weight_training

Sports Medicine Australia 2008, *Safety guidelines for children and young people in sport and recreation*, Australian Government Department of Health and Ageing, http://sma.org.au/wp-content/uploads/2009/05/childrensafetyguidelines-fulldoc.pdf

St John Ambulance 2006, *Australian first aid*, 4th edn, St John Ambulance Australia.

Stafford, I 2011, *Coaching children in sport*, Routledge, New York.

Vrljic, K & Mallet, C 2008, 'Coaching knowledge in identifying football talent', *International Journal of Coaching Science*, vol. 2, no. 1, pp. 63–81.

World Health Organization 2010, 'Childhood overweight and obesity', *Global strategy on diet, physical activity and health*, www.who.int/dietphysicalactivity/childhood/en/

FURTHER READING

Chapter One: Improving children's motor skill development

Australian Council for Health, Physical Education and Recreation 2008, *Fundamental motor skills module*, ACHPER Victorian Branch, Kew East.

Gallahue, D & Ozmun, J 2005, *Understanding motor development: infants, children, adolescents*, 6th edn, McGraw-Hill, New York.

Miah, A & Rich, E 2006, 'Genetic tests for ability?: talent identification and the value of an open future', *Sport, Education & Society*, vol. 11, no. 3, pp. 259–73.

Phillips, E, Keith, D, Renshaw, I & Portus, M 2010, 'Expert performance in sport and the dynamics of talent development', *Sports Medicine*, vol. 40, no. 4, pp. 271–84.

Williams, M & Hodges, N 2004, *Skill acquisition in sport: research, theory and practice*, Routledge, London.

Chapter Two: Tailoring children's exercise to cater for their physical and social development

Laker, A (ed.) 2001, *Developing personal, social and moral education through physical education: a practical guide for teachers*, Routledge, London.

MedicineNet.com (n.d.), *Growth plate injuries*, www.medicinenet.com/growth_plate_fractures_and_injuries/article.htm

Training Science (n.d.), *How does a foundational myth become sacred scientific dogma? The case of AV Hill and the anaerobiosis controversy*, http://trainingscience.net/?page_id=530

Tvisha, P & Gareth, S 2011, 'Influence of intensity of physical activity on adiposity and cardiorespiratory fitness in 5–18 year olds', *Sports Medicine*, vol. 41, no. 6, pp. 477–88.

Vincente-Rodriguez, G 2006, 'How does exercise affect bone development during growth?', *Sports Medicine* , vol. 36, no. 7, pp. 561–9.

Chapter Three: Designing effective training programs

American College of Sports Medicine (n.d.), *Plyometric training for children and adolescents*, ACSM, Indianapolis, Indiana, www.acsm.org/docs/current-comments/plyometrictraining.pdf

Bull, S 2001, *Adherence issues in sport and exercise*, John Wiley & Sons, Oxford.

Dunn, J & Leitschuh, C 2010, *Specialized physical education: adapted, individualized, developmental*, 9th edn, Kendall/Hunt, Dubuque, Indiana.

Chapter Four: Coach communication and athlete development strategies

Kidman, L & McKenzie, A, 1998, *Your kids, their game: a guide for parents, caregivers, teachers and coaches involved in sport*, Australian Sports Commission, Camberra.

Langford, S, 2007, *Sports Commission wants to end ugly parent and ref rage*, media release, Australian Sports Commission, Camberra, 30 May, http://fulltext. ausport.gov.au/fulltext/2007/ascmedia/07.05.30.asp

Chapter Five: Sports psychology for coaching children

Cohn, P 2010, 'These sports kids are prone to emotional tantrums', *The ultimate sports parent*, 1 March, www.youthsportspsychology.com/youth_sports_ psychology_blog/?p=375

Karageorghis, C & Terry, P 2011, *Inside sport psychology*, Human Kinetics, Champaign, Illinois.

Morris, T & Summers, J 2004, *Sport psychology theory, applications and issues*, 2nd edn, John Wiley and Sons, Milton, Queensland.

Van Raalte, J & Brewer, B 2008, *Exploring sport and exercise psychology*, 2nd edn, American Psychological Association, Washington, DC.

Yamine, E 2011, 'Exercise with boys making girls fatter', *Daily Telegraph*, 22 November.

Chapter Six: Sports nutrition for children

AIS Sports Nutrition 2009, *Caffeine: supplement overview*, Australian Sports Commission, Camberra, www.ausport.gov.au/ais/nutrition/supplements/ old_pages/supplement_fact_sheets/group_a_supplements/caffeine

Australian Sports Commission (n.d.), 'Athletes failing to hydrate', *Sports Coach*, vol. 29, no. 2.

Australian Sports Commission (n.d.), 'Pre-event nutrition', *Sports Coach*, vol. 28, no. 3.

Australian Sports Commission (n.d.), 'Supplements in sports—Why are they so tempting?' www.ausport.gov.au/ais/nutrition/supplements/supplements_ in_sport

Dunford, M 2006, *Sports nutrition*, 4th edn, American Dietetic Association.

Ford, R 2008, 'Eat right, learn right', *Teacher: the national education magazine*, no. 195, October, pp. 28–9.

Reaburn, P (n.d.), 'Theory to practice: stomach upsets, sports drinks and team sports', *Sports Coach*, vol. 28, no. 1.

Savino, F, Bonfante, G & Madon, E 1999, 'Use of natural vitamin supplements in children during convalescence and in children with athletic activities', *Minerva Pediatrica*, vol. 51, nos 1–2, pp. 1–9.

Sports Dieticians Australia 2009, *Fact sheet: creatine supplementation and sports performance*, SDA, South Melbourne, April, www.sportsdietitians.com.au/resources/upload/Template%20Creatine%20supplementation%20and%20sports%20performance.pdf

Tysoe, J & Wilson, C 2010, 'Influences of the family and childcare food environments on preschoolers' healthy eating', *Australasian Journal of Early Childhood*, vol. 35, no. 3, pp. 105–14.

Watson, C 2010, 'Evidence suggests extra vitamins can cause problems for children', *Herald Sun*, 31 August, www.heraldsun.com.au/news/victoria/evidence-suggests-extra-vitamins-could-cause-problems-for-children/story-e6frf7l6-1225912053104

Chapter Seven: Caring for and preventing injuries

Cross, T 2007, 'Sports injuries in children', *Medicine Today*, vol. 8, no. 6, pp. 32–41.

Kennedy, D & Fitzgerald, P 1989, *The children's sports injuries handbook*, Bay Books, Kensington, New South Wales.

PureHealthMD (n.d.), 'Child athletes and overuse syndromes', *Discovery fit and health*, Discovery Communications, http://health.howstuffworks.com/wellness/diet-fitness/information/child-athletes-and-overuse-syndromes1.htm

Shanmugam, C & Maffulli, N 2008, 'Sports injuries in children', *British Medical Bulletin*, vol. 86, pp. 33–57.

General information

Bailey, R & Kirk, D 2009, *The Routledge physical education reader*, Routledge, New York.

Doherty, J & Brennan, P 2008, *Physical education and development 3–11: a guide for teachers*, Routledge, London.

Konukman, F, Agbuğa, B, Erdoğan, S, Zorba, E, Demirhan, G & Yılmaz, I 2010, 'Teacher–coach role conflict in school-based physical education in USA: a literature review and suggestions for the future', *Biomedical Human Kinetics*, vol. 2, pp. 19–24.

Krasner, N & Thomas, P 2004, 'Children in sports', University College, London, www.ppt2txt.com/sppt_msc-sports.html

Lynch, J 2001, *Creative coaching*, Human Kinetics, Champaign, Illinois.

Pickup, I & Price, L 2007, *Teaching physical education in the primary school*, Continuum, New York.

Riley, J & Van Rooy, W 2007, 'Perceptions about health in primary school children', *Teaching Science*, vol. 53, no. 4, pp. 32–5.

Wilmore, J, Costill, D & Kenney, W 2008, *Physiology of sport and exercise*, 4th edn, Human Kinetics, Champaign, Illinois.